# ETHNICITY, EQUALITY OF OPPORTUNITY AND THE BRITISH NATIONAL HEALTH SERVICE

# Ethnicity, Equality of Opportunity and the British National Health Service

PAUL IGANSKI
*Department of Sociology, University of Essex*

DAVID MASON
*Department of Sociology, University of Plymouth*

Routledge
Taylor & Francis Group
LONDON AND NEW YORK

First published 2002 by Ashgate Publishing

Reissued 2018 by Routledge
2 Park Square, Milton Park, Abingdon, Oxon OX14 4RN
711 Third Avenue, New York, NY 10017, USA

*Routledge is an imprint of the Taylor & Francis Group, an informa business*



A Library of Congress record exists under LC control number: 2001098005

ISBN 13: 978-1-138-72873-8 (hbk)
ISBN 13: 978-1-315-19039-6 (ebk)

# Contents

# List of Figures and Tables

# 1 Introduction

This book explores the provision of equal employment opportunities in the British National Health Service (NHS). As we shall see, despite sustained exhortation to improvement, and repeated high profile national policy statements and initiatives, there is evidence of long-standing racism in NHS employment practices. At the same time, there is little convincing evidence of systematic attempts to implement nationally developed commitments at the local level; that is, where health care is delivered. The central section of the book draws from a research project commissioned by the English National Board for Nursing, Midwifery and Health Visiting (ENB), carried out between 1996 and 1998 (Iganski *et al.*, 1998),[1] on the recruitment and retention of members of minority ethnic groups into training for nursing, midwifery and health visiting.

Our discussion of the findings of this research is placed in the context of a wider consideration of racial exclusion and equal opportunities in the NHS. Given that nurses represent the largest occupational group in the Service, and are also those most closely involved in the day to day care of patients, their experience arguably has implications for recruitment and selection practices in the NHS more widely. In addition to highlighting such wider practical lessons from the research findings, we also seek to place our discussion of policy questions in the context of a conceptual interrogation of key arguments and debates about equal opportunities and of ethnic difference.

## Terminology

Before proceeding, it is important to clarify the terms that we use in this book. The term 'minority ethnic group' (and its counterpart 'ethnic minority'), while widely used in policy and lay discussions, is not self-evidently unambiguous. It has, moreover, frequently been contested on both intellectual and political grounds. While it is widely understood in Britain to denote a category of people whose recent origins lie in the countries of the New Commonwealth and Pakistan, which groups should be included, and how they should be distinguished and designated, remains a matter of considerable debate. In practice, the criterion which identifies those to whom the term normally refers is having a skin which is not 'white' (what, in the United States, would be designated 'visible minorities'). One consequence of this is that 'ethnic minorities' are treated in many discussions as an undifferentiated category, with characteristics and experiences in common that differentiate them sharply from the rest of the population (compare the discussions in Ballard, 1992; Field, 1987; Modood, 1988; 1990; 1992. See also the discussion in Chapter 7 below). In addition, the important differences between the experiences of men and women are also frequently overlooked (Anthias and Yuval-Davis, 1992). This usage also tends to underplay the increasing diversity of experience of members of different groups (see Modood *et al.*, 1997 and Chapter 7 below).[2]

Despite these problems and the intellectual reservations to which they inevitably give rise, we were constrained in our research design both by the research brief and the form in which data were available. These data themselves reflect prior decisions about which patterns of difference merit measurement and these, in turn, reflect the patterns of disadvantage (and discrimination) which are known, or thought, to characterise the experience of different groups. In this context it should be noted that increasing concerns about the apparent under-representation of some groups in the nursing workforce coincided with the initiation of ethnic monitoring of applications and admissions to nursing, midwifery and health visiting education.

The data available to the research team were contained in the admissions database of the Nurses and Midwives Central Clearing House (NMCCH). These data record the self-classification of applicants in terms of the ethnic group categories used in the 1991 Census:

White
Black - Caribbean, Black - African, Black - Other (please describe)
Indian, Pakistani, Bangladeshi, Chinese
Any other ethnic group (please describe)

To these, the NMCCH added an 'Irish' category in 1994.[3]

In what follows, the term minority ethnic group is deployed in a way that reflects the conventional usage discussed above and the constraints of the data available. As in Census derived data, members of minority ethnic groups are, then, deemed to be those who have classified themselves in terms of one of the ethnic categories other than 'white'. It should be noted, however, that we have preferred the term 'minority ethnic group' to 'ethnic minority' in order to emphasise the plurality of groupings involved and to encourage a recognition of the diversity of experience characteristic of the groups in question.

## Methods and Data Sources

The ENB commissioned research, the findings of which we explore below, aimed to:

- map the national pattern of applications, from members of minority ethnic groups, to pre- and post-registration nursing, midwifery and health visiting courses;
- identify the ratios of applications to offers of places, and of these to rates of acceptance, among members of different ethnic groups;
- investigate recruitment and selection practices;
- use the evidence accumulated to advise the ENB on the future development of equal opportunities policy.

For the analysis of applications to pre-registration training we used data provided by the ENB covering all applications made through the Nurses and Midwives Central Clearing House (NMCCH) between 1993 and 1996. We present the results of our analysis in Chapter 4. The material presented in the chapter updates our earlier reports (Iganski *et al.*, 1998; Iganski *et al.*, 1999) as it incorporates more recent data from the Nurses and Midwives Admissions Service (NMAS) covering applications from 1997 to 2000. We discuss both data sets in more detail in Chapter 4. We had originally hoped to conduct a comparable analysis in respect of post-registration training. However, no nationally compiled data were available at the time of the research commissioned by the ENB, or since.

We had two broad areas of concern for the research into recruitment and selection practices. First, we were interested in evaluating whether selection processes used by nurse education and training institutions had incorporated equal opportunity policy guidance offered by the ENB and by other bodies like the King's Fund Equal Opportunities Task Force. Second, we were interested in whether nurse education and training institutions specifically targeted minority ethnic groups in their recruitment measures, and if they did, what could be learnt from their activities. These research aims suggested an in-depth qualitative approach, as the goal was to learn from and to be able to evaluate, recruitment and selection policies and practices. We therefore needed to establish a clear understanding of how recruitment and selection actually worked in practice.

The ideal research strategy would have been to observe at first hand recruitment and selection processes in action. However, even if it were possible for us to observe all the processes themselves - and it is questionable whether we could have been present at all of the activities involved - such a strategy would be highly resource intensive. The next best approach was to use individuals, who occupy key roles in regard to the policies and practices, as informants. In effect, such an approach involves an ethnography of the policy process, whereby the researchers construct an understanding through the perspectives of the key actors involved. Whilst informants each have their own particular perspectives, commonly bounded by the role they play in the policy processes, the strategy enabled us to put together a picture by validating one respondent's perspectives against another's. This strategy is also resource intensive due to the length of discussions needed with key informants and the number of individuals commonly involved in recruitment and selection activities who might appropriately serve as key informants.

Working to the resource constraints of the project, our investigation of recruitment and selection processes was carried out in eight nurse education and training institutions. We discuss how we selected these institutions in Chapter 5. Each institution served as a case study, as we constructed an understanding of the processes at work in each of the institutions separately, although in this book, and in our earlier reports, the findings from the institutions are combined into an aggregated account. This approach to presenting the research findings was thought to be necessary to ensure the anonymity of the case study institutions and individual respondents. Conscious of the sensitivity of the issues under investigation and of the harm that could be done to the careers of respondents by careless research design or reporting, we took great care to preserve individual anonymity and confidentiality. Nurse education centres are referred to only by pseudonyms and, with the exception of one case of good practice, care has been taken to present the research findings in aggregated form, rather than as case studies of each institution. Respondents were fully briefed about the nature and purposes of the research and were given an unconditional right to withdraw at any stage. Most of our interviews were tape-recorded - with the respondent's permission - and the tapes transcribed by a transcription service which was asked to sign a confidentiality agreement.

As discussed above, we had two broad areas of concern for the investigation of recruitment and selection practices. First, we were concerned to discover whether selection processes utilised were consistent with equal opportunities good practice. Second, we were interested in whether nurse education and training institutions specifically targeted minority ethnic groups in their recruitment measures, and if they did, what could be learnt from their activities. Different data collection and analysis strategies were applied to the two areas of investigation. In order to investigate selection policy and practice, the Heads of each of the eight case study centres, together with the senior managers with overall responsibility for selection in the centres, were first asked to 'talk the interviewers through' the processes by which applicants are selected for training. The aim was deductively to evaluate whether the processes used by the institutions had incorporated the policy guidance offered by bodies like the King's Fund Equal Opportunities Task Force and whether there were areas of selection practice where there was the potential for unfair practice or discrimination to occur. Our lines of enquiry are discussed in detail in Chapter 5, but, in outline, we asked about selection criteria, procedures for shortlisting and interviewing, the training provided to staff involved in the selection processes, and the monitoring of selection decisions. The various elements of equal opportunity policy guidance provided a checklist for the topics covered in the discussions. The data were also analysed deductively with the elements providing an analytic structure and a format for the presentation of the findings in Chapter 5.

For the investigation of recruitment measures, our second broad area of concern, we applied a different research style from that used in the investigation of recruitment practices. We used a grounded theory approach to the collection of data and to the data analysis (although it was in a modified form as we discuss in Chapter 6). Such an approach suggested itself from the research objectives. A prime objective was to learn from the experience of the case study institutions. A grounded theory approach is suitable to that objective as a fundamental principle of the approach is to generate 'theory' that is grounded in empirical data through an inductive process, rather than establishing *a priori* concepts or hypotheses that are subsequently explored or tested through the data (Glaser and Strauss, 1967). An inductive approach was suggested by the research objectives as, to learn from the experience of the institutions, we needed to develop an understanding of the complexity of processes - such as the antecedents, barriers, constraints, facilitators - behind the establishment and implementation of recruitment initiatives.

A grounded theory approach does not, however, imply that researchers can approach their data with a *tabula rasa* (Glaser and Strauss, 1967: 3), and that a 'pure' inductive analysis can be applied to the data (Pidgeon, 1996: 82). Researchers approach their data with their own initial perspectives (Charmaz, 1990), pre-conceptions and assumptions which will inevitably influence the questions that are asked and the interpretations made of the data collected. As the aim, though, is for the emergent ideas to be grounded in the data, and for authenticity of the ideas in relation to the experience of the researched, it is incumbent upon researchers to explore their potential biases and pre-conceptions and, where some are maintained and influence data collection and analysis, to make them explicit. The chief assumption with which we approached this project was derived directly from the original research specification provided by the ENB. This made explicit the link between patterns of ethnic representation and the formulation and implementation of equal opportunities policy. The implication is that, where under-representation exists, nurse education and training institutions *should* take active measures to recruit students from black and Asian minority ethnic groups for training in nursing and midwifery. The case for such measures is discussed in Chapter 3 of this book. This assumption meant that we did not set out initially to seek the views of the research respondents about whether targeted recruitment was desirable as a basis for deciding whether to ask about any recruitment initiatives. Instead, respondents were asked about recruitment initiatives first, then subsequently about their desirability, in an attempt to gauge the level of commitment to the initiatives. The difference may be subtle but nevertheless significant, as the prime goal was not to investigate desirability of the initiatives *per se* by using a large portion of the interview time exploring respondents' views about the matter. Instead, the aim was to use the time exploring the respondents' experience to find ideas for targeting that could be disseminated to other institutions.

## Background

The ENB's research specification made explicit a link between the representation of members of minority ethnic groups, among applicants and entrants to the nursing and midwifery professions, and the formulation and implementation of the Board's equal opportunities policy. The implication was that continued under-representation would constitute *prima facie* evidence of an absence of equality of opportunity and raise questions about the fairness and equity of recruitment and selection procedures. It is important to note that such evidence does not provide conclusive proof that recruitment and selection processes are discriminatory. As we shall see, it is possible that under-representation is a consequence of a range of other processes and influences that lead to a lack of applications from members of some groups. In such circumstances, the point at issue would be less discriminatory selection practices and more a matter of a failure to proactively seek applications from under-represented groups. In the discussions in Chapters 5 and 6 below, we consider each of these questions in the light of the analysis of application and admissions statistics for nursing and midwifery training. As we shall argue in Chapter 7, however, it remains a possibility that under-representation of some groups is a result of differential occupational choice. In point of fact, it would be safe to conclude that this were indeed the explanation only if we could be confident that measures were in place that ensured bias free selection and appropriately targeted minority ethnic communities as potential sources of recruits. In other words, the first requirement would be an effective equal opportunities and positive action strategy, as advocated by the Codes of Practice of the Commission for Racial Equality and the Equal Opportunities Commission (CRE, 1984a; EOC, 1985) and the Employment Department's *Equal Opportunities Ten Point Plan for Employers* (U.K. Employment Department, 1991).

Since the mid-1980s an increasing number of organisations have developed such policies or reviewed and extended earlier programmes. In the public sector, a number of local authorities and public utilities took a leading role while, in the private sector, large-scale employers with established reputations for good employment practice were prominent (Jewson *et al.*, 1995). In the late 1980s, the CRE funded research designed to assess the impact of its Code of Practice on the awareness and behaviour of employers (CRE, 1989). A national survey of 899 employers revealed a very high level of basic awareness about the existence of the Code, although only a quarter had read through or glanced at the text itself. Of the latter, some two-thirds had developed formal, written equal opportunities policies of some kind. Very few indeed, however, had policies that could be regarded as comprehensive or with adequate systems for monitoring their effectiveness. The study also reported on detailed case studies of eight employers who had taken extensive action with respect to equal opportunities. These revealed that where employers committed themselves to policies aimed at eliminating specific obstacles to equal opportunities within their workplaces there had been an increase in the numbers of ethnic minority people recruited and promoted.

However, the study was cautious even in the case of these examples of good practice. In most cases positive effects were confined to the attraction of minority ethnic recruits into lower grades, rather than advancement into middle and senior level positions. Moreover there was frequently said to be an undue emphasis on process rather than outcomes. In contrast, the report argued that the 'ultimate measure' of the success of an equal opportunities policy must be changes in the proportion and distribution of ethnic minority employees throughout the organisation.

In this context, the study identified five stages in the development of effective equal opportunities programmes (1989: 38-9). They constitute a cycle, embodying review and feedback, that policy makers are recommended to follow. The study argued that significant results are not obtained until the fifth stage is reached. The five stages are as follows:

1. Acknowledgement of the need to take action to adopt a policy.
2. Recognition that processes need to be implemented to make policy work (for example, the issue of guidelines to managers involved in recruitment).

3. Recognition of the need for factual information about the effectiveness of policy (for example, through collection and analysis of ethnic monitoring data with respect to applicants and existing employees).
4. Evaluation of factual evidence in order to identify barriers to equal opportunities caused by management practices past and present.
5. Acceptance and adoption of specific measures to remove barriers to equal opportunities at the workplace and to change managers' behaviour within a clear framework of management objectives.

The kinds of measures required to reach the fifth stage are set out in a number of advisory documents perhaps the most comprehensive and influential of which is the Employment Department's *Equal Opportunities Ten Point Plan for Employers* (1991). Two points in the recommended list of actions are of particular significance for this discussion: first, the need to establish an action plan including targets (Point 2) and, second, the establishment of 'positive action' measures, where appropriate, to target, encourage and enhance the recruitment of under-represented groups in the workforce (Point 7).

Prior to our study, there had been no research on the extent to which nurse education centres have implemented equal opportunities measures for the recruitment and selection of applicants. However, an investigation in 1991 of the implementation of equal opportunities policies by Health Authorities and Health Boards across the U.K., using the CRE's five stages as a measure, found that many Health Authorities had only taken tentative steps towards policy implementation in employment more generally (Iganski, 1992). As we shall see, in the nurse education centres studied in our research (as generally in the NHS), there was little evidence of widespread effective policy development, a conclusion borne out by a more recent study commissioned by the ENB (2000). Crucially, moreover, most respondents in our research displayed at best limited appreciation of the arguments for effective provision of this kind (see Chapter 6 below).

Characteristically, two kinds of arguments are adduced in support of equal opportunities measures. They are, respectively, those that appeal to considerations of equity and fairness, and those that rely upon appeals to self-interest. With respect to the first, a lack of equity is typically seen to raise issues of social justice and citizenship that have implications well beyond the boundaries of particular professions or occupations (Jewson and Mason, 1994; Mason and Jewson, 1992). With respect to the second, arguments, often characterised as a 'business case' for equal opportunities, place the issue firmly within the realm of self-interest rather than relying on altruism or justice (U.K. Employment Department, 1991; Jewson and Mason, 1994).

This second set of arguments has come to be particularly influential since the late 1980s among senior policy-makers in the NHS. For instance, on the launch of a *Management Guide* to the implementation of equal employment opportunities policies in the NHS (NHS Training Authority, 1989) the Minister of Health, David Mellor, argued that: 'Equal opportunities is not just about social justice - important though that is. As every good employer well knows, equal opportunities has a more practical dimension, namely securing a future workforce in terms of numbers and quality and making the best use of our most valuable resource - our staff' (U.K. Department of Health, 1989). Nearly three years later David Mellor's successor at the Department of Health, Virginia Bottomley, stated publicly in promoting the *Opportunity 2000* campaign in the NHS that it was 'not a philanthropic exercise ... but enlightened self-interest' (Iganski, 1993a).

In the context of the health service these kinds of arguments have had a number of foci, two of which are of particular relevance to the recruitment of minority ethnic nurses, midwives and health visitors. First, under-representation of some groups is said to have implications for the quality of health care provision to the diverse communities making up modern Britain. Second, given the younger age profiles of some of the groups concerned, their significance as a potential source of labour for nursing and midwifery is greater than would be suggested merely by the total relative size of the communities in question. Each of these issues is discussed in detail in later chapters.

## Organisation of the Book

In Chapter 2 we review evidence about the incidence of racism in the National Health Service. Particular attention is paid to studies of selection for medical school and for training in nursing and midwifery. Data from our own research reveal a widespread belief that perceptions or experiences of racism exercise a disincentive effect on potential applicants from minority ethnic groups.

Chapter 3 considers the history of equal opportunities policy in the NHS to indicate how arguments for enhanced provision have increasingly been framed in terms of enlightened self-interest or a 'business case'.

Chapter 4 returns to the supposed disincentive effect of racism on potential recruits from minority ethnic communities. It reviews earlier arguments anticipating the demise of the 'black nurse' and considers whether the evidence from patterns of application bears out such predictions. In point of fact, our analysis reveals complex patterns of under- and, in some cases, over-representation. While this evidence does not bear out some of the more apocalyptic predictions discussed, the analysis does reveal differential success rates among applicants from different ethnic groups that cannot be easily explained. It suggests that there may be factors at work in selection processes that discriminate in terms of ethnicity and that these may well be concentrated at the shortlisting stage.

Against this background, Chapter 5 presents qualitative data drawn from case studies of eight nurse training institutions. These suggest that, some examples of good practice notwithstanding, there was considerable scope for the intrusion of potentially discriminatory criteria into selection processes, notably at the shortlisting stage.

In Chapter 6 we consider the kinds of measures that might be introduced to increase the pool of minority ethnic applicants to nursing and midwifery. Again drawing on our case study institutions, we show that good practice was fragmentary and generally under-developed. More significantly, the arguments for effective, proactive initiatives were neither well nor widely understood.

Chapter 7 raises a number of questions about how ethnicity is to be conceptualised in the context of conventional equal opportunities arguments. It reviews important evidence about patterns of upward occupational and educational mobility, as well as changes in the patterning of ethnic identities. We also raise some potentially difficult questions about the relationship between exclusionary processes and occupational choice.

Finally, Chapter 8 revisits some of the arguments commonly deployed in support of equal opportunities provision in the context of the evidence presented earlier in the book. In particular, we raise questions about the relationship between moral arguments and those based on self-interest. We also question to what extent the employment equality and service delivery agendas are, in practice, congruent. Concluding that it is important to keep in mind the political character of equal opportunities, we argue that policy development in the health service must transcend individual initiative and responsibility and focus instead on the contribution of the whole health care team. Crucially, we suggest that the capacity of the NHS, as a key national institution, to advance the equality agenda depends on the success of a wider national drive to build a more ethnically inclusive society.

## Notes

1 The research was conducted by the authors jointly with Amanda Spong, Ann Humphreys and Mary Watkins, who co-authored the report to the ENB. Although this book contains a wide range of additional material, our co-researchers must share much of the credit for whatever merits the arguments presented here may have. We alone, of course, are responsible for their deficiencies. We should also like to record our gratitude to Sonia Crow, of the ENB, for her advice and support during the prosecution of the research and to all those respondents who must, of necessity, remain anonymous here. We would also like to thank the members of the research project steering group for their constructive comments on the research; Jeannette Arnold, Nicholas Jewson, Anthony Price, Margaret Redshaw, Angela Senior, and Satnam Virdee. Sarah Azhashemi, of the Nurses and Midwives Clearing House, and Jan Parkin of the NHS Management Executive helpfully provided us with data used in Chapter 4. We are also grateful to Jennifer Galland for assistance with some of the material used in Chapter 2, and Lucinda Platt for a critical reading of an earlier version of Chapter 4.

2 For more extended discussions of these issues see Mason (1991), (1992) and (2000).

3 For a discussion of some of the difficulties of these categories see Chapter 7.

# 2 'Racism' and the British National Health Service

A casual observer may be forgiven for believing that 'racism' has just been discovered in the British National Health Service, on account of the recent claims made about 'institutional racism' in the health services. The report of the Macpherson inquiry (1999) into the racist murder of Stephen Lawrence, published in 1999, thrust the concept of 'institutional racism' in police services firmly onto the public policy agenda. Not long after, an editorial in the *British Medical Journal* (McKenzie, 1999) argued that unless historic processes of discrimination in the health services were addressed, the NHS could similarly be accused of institutional racism. That same year, at the Royal College of Nursing Congress, Christine Hancock, General Secretary of the RCN, accepted that the organisation was also guilty of institutional racism (U.K. House of Commons, 2000). More recently, a collection of essays on *Racism in Medicine* (Coker, 2001), published by the King's Fund - the leading health services 'thinktank', liberally uses the term 'institutional racism' to describe the experience of minority ethnic doctors. The editor of the collection, Naz Coker, argued that: 'No aspect of a doctor's working life is untouched by racism. Discrimination begins in medical schools and affects the whole of a person's career. Harassment and bullying, from both colleagues and patients, are daily facts of life for black and Asian doctors' (Carvel, 2001).

However, even a cursory reading of the literature shows that claims of racism at work in the NHS go back a long way. Writing in the *Nursing Times* in the early 1980s, Protasia Torkington argued that 'Every black professional employed in the National Health Service has experienced racism in one form or another' (Torkington, 1984: 4). Yet allegations of racism were not as readily admitted by NHS management then, and in policy circles, as they perhaps are today. Instead, claims of racism were allegedly met by 'surprise and indignation' (Agbolegbe, 1984: 19) and were rejected by managers who claimed that all the evidence was 'anecdotal, exaggerated and impressionistic' (Alibhai, 1988: 27). The presence of large numbers of black and other minority ethnic staff in the NHS was even allegedly held up as evidence that discrimination did not occur (Pearson, 1987: 25). We observe too, in Chapter 3 of this book, that such a view was held by officials in the then Department of Health and Social Security in the early 1980s. After all, the National Health Service has actively recruited migrant workers, and it has historically been the largest single employer of people from the black and Asian minority ethnic groups in the U.K. Might this not indicate equality of opportunity at work?

It does not mean, however, that health service workers from minority ethnic communities are represented across the full range of occupational functions or that they have access to genuine equality of opportunity. As the Commission for Racial Equality has noted, there have been a substantial number of industrial tribunal cases in which Health Authorities have been found to have unlawfully discriminated against employees or job applicants. Also, according to the CRE, 'as numerous reports have shown, there are still many, often glaring disparities between white and ethnic minority employees in terms of training and career opportunities, grade and specialism' (1991: 6). Added to this, there is a vast amount of anecdotal evidence concerning discrimination at work.

As is the practice today, the NHS has in the past actively recruited overseas labour - particularly for the nursing and ancillary sectors - due to periods of shortfall in the numbers of indigenous British workers prepared to work in the health services. Black migrant workers - and especially black women - have consequently made a significant contribution in the shape of their labour power to the British National Health Service since its foundation. However, their experience has been characterised by subordination and exploitation, rather than equity with their white colleagues (Alibhai, 1988: 26). In the case of nurses, for instance, anecdotal evidence suggests that having been recruited to low-paid work, many migrant women were subject to exclusionary processes that maintained them in positions of disadvantage. As we discuss later in this chapter, such experience has arguably served as a deterrent to the pursuit of a career in nursing by subsequent generations of women from Britain's minority ethnic communities.

There are a number of indicators of systematic inequality at work. Historically, there has been a tendency for minority ethnic staff to be concentrated in semi- and unskilled work such as in the ancillary and maintenance sectors. Moreover, even though they have a strong presence in the skilled occupations of nursing and medicine, they have been concentrated in the lower reaches of those professions. It is not possible to determine the full extent of occupational segregation by ethnic group for the NHS as a whole as national data are incomplete, but research evidence over time indicates consistent patterns of inequality at work. There was early evidence of such inequality in the case of migrant nurses. The Newsletter of the Institute of Race Relations in 1968 reported that 'Commonwealth' nurses were under-represented amongst senior nursing staff despite the fact that as a group they had been working in the NHS long enough to achieve a greater representation amongst senior nurses than was apparent. It was observed that one suggestion, 'offered (privately) as to the lack of promotion, in the case of West Indians in particular, was that they are "too slow, less qualified and less able to take charge" ... if such bias is widespread in the nursing profession it would go far in explaining the lack of promotion for overseas-born nurses' (Gish, 1968: 458).

Over ten years later, in the case of Whittington hospital in London in 1979, Doyal *et al.* observed that nurses of Afro-Caribbean origin were found to be under-represented in the senior grades of ward sister and above in comparison to their representation amongst the more junior level of staff nurses and nursery nurses. In contrast, nurses of Irish origin were over-represented at senior level. Afro-Caribbeans were also over-represented among the lower grades of SEN and pupil nurses, and also amongst nursing auxiliaries (Doyal *et al.*, 1980: 83-84). Similarly, data provided by Macquisten (1986) on the ethnic composition of the nursing workforce in Southern Derbyshire Health Authority in the mid 1980s indicated that Afro-Caribbean nurses were under-represented amongst senior nurses.

There is similar evidence of systematic disadvantage for minority ethnic groups affecting Administrative, Clerical, and Senior Managerial Staff (Iganski, 1993b: 53) and doctors (Anwar and Ali, 1987; McNaught, 1988: 40; Ward, 1993). In the case of doctors, one of the earliest studies of overseas doctors in the National Health Service was carried out by the Policy Studies Institute in the late 1970s. It found that over a fifth (22 per cent) of 'coloured doctors' believed that they had been unsuccessful in applications for hospital positions because of 'race' discrimination (Smith, 1980: 138). A later survey of overseas doctors in one Regional Health Authority in the 1980s, published by the Commission for Racial Equality (Anwar and Ali, 1987), reported that large proportions of both white (40 per cent) and 'ethnic minority' doctors (52 per cent) believed that 'overseas' doctors were discriminated against in their region. Some believed that 'overseas' doctors were less likely to get jobs in the popular hospitals and specialities, and approximately a quarter of both white and 'ethnic minority' doctors believed that if two equally qualified doctors applied for a post, the white doctor would be successful. Approximately one tenth of overseas doctors believed that this would occur even if the overseas applicant was more qualified than the white applicant. The study also observed patterns of inequality across the medical hierarchy, as 67 per cent of white British trained doctors in the survey were at consultant grade, compared to 36 per cent of those trained overseas, and 30 per cent of minority ethnic doctors trained in Britain. Overseas doctors were also just short of being numerically dominant in the two least popular specialities of Geriatrics and Psychiatry.

Neither perceived experience, nor belief in discrimination at work, provide evidence of actual discrimination. However, unequivocal evidence of racial discrimination in the labour market has been provided over time by a series of experimental investigations (Daniel, 1968; Jowell and Prescott-Clarke, 1970; McIntosch and Smith, 1974; Hubbuck and Carter, 1980; Firth, 1981; Brown and Gay, 1985). One of these types of investigation famously exposed discrimination against minority ethnic doctors. Esmail and Everington (1993) sent pairs of applications, one with an English name and one with an Asian name, but matched in terms of other characteristics relevant to the applications, for twenty-three advertised house officer posts in non-teaching hospitals. Neither of the pair was shortlisted for eleven of the posts. The applicant with the English name was shortlisted for each of the remaining twelve posts, but the Asian applicant was only shortlisted in six of them. Even on the basis of a small number of applications this is clear evidence of discrimination at work. Esmail and Everington would have sent matched applications for further posts, but their arrest by the Fraud Squad put a stop to the research.

## Selection of Students for Medical School

Despite the evidence of employment discrimination discussed above, research evidence concerning discrimination against minority ethnic groups in selection for training in the health services professions is limited.

However, there is arguably more evidence in the case of entry to medical training than entry to the other professions. The evidence has recently been reviewed elsewhere (Esmail, 2001) but it is instructive to discuss it briefly here as it highlights areas of the selection process that are potentially vulnerable to discrimination. We focus on those areas in some detail in this book in the case of selection to training in nursing and midwifery. Minority ethnic students, and Asian students in particular, are over-represented in medical schools compared with the representation of the groups concerned in the population as a whole (Esmail, 2001). However, this does not indicate the absence of discrimination.

An investigation for the Commission for Racial Equality into selection practices at St George's medical school in the late 1980s produced unequivocal evidence of discrimination (CRE, 1988a). The investigation strengthened suspicions arising from earlier research into the selection of applicants to medical school (cf. McManus and Richards, 1985; Collier and Burke, 1986). This was especially so as the high proportion of minority ethnic students at St. George's relative to other schools might have provided grounds to believe that discrimination was not occurring there, or at least that there was less discrimination.

In the St George's case the CRE observed that discrimination was written into a computer program used to shortlist applicants. The program was intended to mimic selection decisions made over a number of years. 'Non-Caucasian' and female applicants were given a negative weighting by the program. The effect was that for the academic year 1985-1986, the Commission estimated that 57 applicants were denied an interview due to the discrimination written into the program. For earlier years, for which records were no longer available, the Commission's best estimate was that approximately 60 applicants were similarly denied an interview each year. The Commission also noted that, following interview, there was a statistically significant difference between the proportions of 'Caucasian' and 'non-Caucasian' applicants offered medical school places, that was not due to their relative ranking at shortlisting. In the absence of records concerning the reasons for rejection following interview, the Commission was not able to conclude that discrimination had occurred at interview, but an earlier investigation (McManus and Richards, 1985) indicates what might have been happening. Judgements made during shortlisting were analysed for applicants to St. Mary's medical school in 1981. It was observed that U.K. nationals with non-European surnames were more likely to be determined on the strength of their application forms as being unsuitable on non-academic criteria such as 'interests' and 'contribution to the community'. A smaller proportion of them were interviewed, and following interview those with non-European surnames were again more likely to be assessed as being unsuitable on non-academic criteria, even though they were assessed as having equivalent academic ability to those with European surnames. Clearly, the less objective the selection criteria, the greater the potential for bias to distort selection decisions. We return to this in more detail below in discussing the selection of applicants for training in nursing and midwifery.

More recent research has also provided indications of discrimination in the selection process. In 1995 Esmail and colleagues published a league table of medical schools – in the *British Medical Journal* – of the likelihood of 'white' applicants, compared with minority ethnic applicants, being accepted when controlling for A-level grades. The data provided prima facie evidence of discrimination as in the great majority of medical schools white applicants were more likely to be accepted (Esmail *et al.*, 1995). However, the most comprehensive research to date involved an analysis of data provided by the Universities and Colleges Admissions Service (UCAS) on applications to medical schools in 1996 and 1997 (McManus, 1998). In controlling for other confounding variables, McManus observed that applicants from minority ethnic groups, and male applicants, were disadvantaged in that they were less likely to receive an offer of a place than other applicants. According to McManus 'it seems reasonable to conclude that in some cases at some schools discrimination is occurring, wittingly or unwittingly. Direct discrimination seems unlikely (but not impossible), although an aberrant minority of selectors may be subverting an otherwise fair system' (1998: 1114). In addition to suggesting that indirect discrimination may be operating in the assessment of candidates' likely academic attainment from estimated A-level grades, McManus suggested that indirect discrimination may arise 'from assessing motivational and personality factors indirectly through achievements and experiences with different meanings in different cultural groups' (1998: 1114-15). In light of the research findings the Council of Heads of Medical Schools (CHMS) issued an action plan, following consultation with the Commission for Racial Equality, aimed at ensuring openness and fairness in the selection of medical students (CHMS press release 15/10/1998). As part of the plan each medical school was expected to review its academic and non-academic selection criteria.

## Entry into Nursing and Midwifery Training

In the 1970s and 1980s it was controversially alleged that many migrant women who applied to train as nurses in the NHS were channelled by deception to the bottom of the nursing hierarchy where they served as cheap labour (Black Women's Group, 1974: 226; Ramdin, 1987: 310). One of the ways this allegedly occurred was that some applicants were promised entry to professional nurse training to become State Registered Nurses (SRN), but once they arrived in Britain that promise was broken as they were employed as auxiliary nurses without any guarantees of access to training. Torkington (1987) provided the account of one nurse who claimed that the matron of the hospital where she worked even contrived to keep her there as a nursing auxiliary by sabotaging her applications to other hospitals for SRN training (Torkington, 1987: 27).

There is also anecdotal evidence of migrant nurses being channelled into the lower grade pupil nurse training for the SEN qualification that limited career prospects to the lowest levels of the nursing hierarchy. Disproportionate numbers of black migrant nurses were recruited to train as SENs rather than as SRNs, and it has been argued that this practice continued for overseas nurses up until the early 1980s (Hicks, 1982: 789). Until the recent movement towards the introduction of a single system of training for nurses, there were two distinct levels of qualification: the State Enrolled Nurse and the State Registered Nurse. The former was of lower status and typically enjoyed fewer opportunities for promotion to more senior positions. Evidence suggests that nurses of minority ethnic origin were markedly over-represented among SENs (Doyal *et al.*, 1980; Torkington, 1987; Pearson, 1987; Baxter, 1988; Iganski, 1993b; Ward, 1993). It appears that some of the migrant women were channelled into SEN training unwittingly (Torkington, 1987: 27) through the attraction of a shorter training course in comparison to SRN training (Black Women's Group, 1974: 227) and many did not know that two tiers of training existed (Pearson, 1987: 25-26; Baxter, 1988: 25). Others who did not have the educational qualifications required for entry to SRN training appear not to have been given the same opportunity as white British women to sit an entry test instead (Hicks, 1982: 789). For many of the migrant women SEN training was unrecognised in their countries of origin and it was therefore worthless if they wanted to return. Some of the nurses have reported that they felt isolated when they realised their dilemma as they got little support from their schools of nursing and colleagues in trying to alter their career path (Baxter, 1988: 26). One black nurse recalled that the pupil nurses - who in the hospital in which she worked appeared to be mostly black - were treated as 'just a pair of hands'. They were given the unpleasant jobs on the ward whilst actual training in nursing procedures was given to the mostly white student nurses (Hicks, 1982: 789). Black migrant nurses were also allegedly channelled into the less popular specialities and less prestigious nursing schools, and it was even argued in 1982 that this practice was still continuing (Hicks, 1982: 790). In short, it has been argued that on the ward floor, black women serviced the patients, the professional nurses (SRNs) and the doctors (Black Women's Group, 1974: 227).

*Pre-Registration Training*

Despite the anecdotal evidence of discrimination discussed above, the only published research investigation of the experience of minority ethnic applicants for pre-registration training, prior to our own research which we report in this book, was carried out by the Commission for Racial Equality in 1986 (CRE, 1987). The research used a mail questionnaire sent to thirty-two schools of nursing in England and Wales, with thirty returned. From the limited data collected it was evident that student nurses from the black and Asian minority ethnic groups were under-represented amongst trainees compared with their representation in the population as a whole. They were also, as a group, less successful in their applications, compared with whites. A variety of potentially contributory factors were identified. Some nurse training schools set entry criteria above the minimum educational qualifications required for entry and this may have disadvantaged and deterred some applicants from the minority ethnic groups. The most common methods of recruitment were by word of mouth (which has been shown to disadvantage the minority ethnic groups when they are already under-represented in a workforce [CRE, 1982]) and unsolicited letters which may also rely on 'inside knowledge' of vacancies. The CRE also observed that, in addition to the use of educational qualifications, selectors evaluated candidates on the basis of a range of non-academic qualities. The most common were 'motivation', and 'interest in the caring profession' and were evaluated by a number of schools on the basis of the candidate's involvement in voluntary work of a caring nature. More subjective criteria were also applied, such as; 'emotional stability', 'intelligence', 'imagination', and 'ability to integrate without undue difficulty'. It is not difficult to see how such subjective criteria are susceptible to the intrusion of, perhaps unwittingly, biased judgements (compare the discussion in Jenkins, 1986). In commenting on the research findings, the Principal of the Commission for Racial Equality's employment division observed that a stereotypical conception of the ideal applicant for nurse training is of a white middle-class female. He concluded that: 'If that stereotype looms large in the minds of selectors - and one gets the feeling it perhaps does - that is something that needs to be looked at very hard because certainly that will militate against ethnic minority groups' (Cole, 1987: 30).

To avoid such bias in selection decisions, the CRE has recommended that: 'staff responsible for shortlisting, interviewing and selecting candidates should be ... given guidance or training on the effects which generalised assumptions and prejudices about race can have on selection decisions ... (and) ... made aware of the possible misunderstandings that can occur in interviews between persons of different cultural background' (CRE, 1984a: para. 1.14b). With regard to recruitment and selection generally, the King's Fund Equal Opportunities Task Force recommended in 1987 that 'everybody involved in the recruitment and selection of staff should receive recruitment and selection training within six months of their appointment, or within two years of the adoption of an equal opportunities policy' (KFEOTF, 1987: 9). We return to these recommendations in Chapter 5 of this book.

There is also anecdotal evidence of some minority ethnic groups being steered away from nursing in careers guidance provided within schools. For example Baxter (1988), in interviews with a purposive sample of 33 respondents, found evidence of the stereotyping of minority ethnic groups. Thus, young Asian women were discouraged from pursuing nursing as a career on the basis of supposed incompatibility between the nursing uniform and stereotypes about cultural dress styles. They were steered instead into occupations demanding higher academic qualifications. By contrast, African-Caribbean women were allegedly advised on the basis of stereotypical assumptions that nursing would be an appropriate career for them (Baxter, 1988: 31-32).

*Post-Registration Training*

Issues of equality of opportunity and the recruitment of nurses and midwives have arguably been the focus of more research and investigation in the case of post-registration than of pre-registration training. The research, though, has been limited and has focused on the activities of health service employers, rather than nurse education and training institutions. In the late 1980s the Commission for Racial Equality (CRE, 1988b) carried out a formal investigation into promotion practices in South Manchester District Health Authority. Although suspicions of unlawful discrimination were not proved, the investigation revealed that qualified 'black' nurses felt they were unfairly treated with regard to further training. From their interviews with staff, the Commission observed that black and white staff were equally likely to report that they had been on managerial training but black staff were less likely to report that they had attended 'other training' which they felt was relevant to promotion.

Data collected for the investigation revealed that black staff spent fewer days on non-statutory training courses than the refresher courses which they were obliged to attend, whilst the opposite was the case for white staff. The patterns of applications for the two groups of staff also differed. Whilst black and white staff were equally likely to have applied at least once for training, the latter were likely to have made a significantly greater number of applications. Some black staff felt that this was because they were not encouraged to attend training courses as often as whites.

Anecdotal evidence of inequity was also provided by Baxter's interviews (1988). Some minority ethnic staff working in what they believed to be less popular specialities reported that they encountered barriers to training for transfer into higher status and more popular areas of work (Baxter, 1988: 34-6).

More recent and comprehensive research appears to support the earlier evidence. Beishon *et al.* (1995), in research commissioned by the NHS Management Executive and carried out by the Policy Studies Institute, report from a mail survey of respondent nurses and midwives, that most minority ethnic, but not white, nursing and midwifery staff believed that racial discrimination operated in the allocation of training opportunities across the NHS and to a lesser extent in their own workplaces. In addition, approximately one quarter of black and Asian minority ethnic nurses and midwives in the survey believed that they had been personally discriminated against in the provision of training opportunities.

From case studies of six health service employers, Beishon *et al.* (1995) identified two broad recruitment channels to post-registration training. In the first, individuals become aware of a training opportunity and informally approach their manager, with final approval given by the senior nurse of the specialty. Beishon *et al.* found that in their six case study employers post-registration courses were advertised to nursing staff either by a booklet setting out the courses for the coming year, or by circulars (1995: 80). However, in the light of the evidence of differential access to training opportunities, and suspicions of unlawful discrimination, the King's Fund Equal Opportunities Task Force recommended that all 'staff should be counselled individually to provide advice about training requirements for promotion' (KFEOTF, 1990: 22). The Task Force also recommended that 'the application process should be made clear to all staff', and that training opportunities should be widely advertised so that all staff are fully aware of them (KFEOTF, 1990: 22).

A second channel of recruitment to post-registration training, identified by Beishon *et al.*, entails managers identifying career development needs of individual staff and advising them to apply (1995: 77-78). Since it relies upon relationships between individual managers and staff, however, such a system is, in principle, vulnerable to the intrusion of personal biases unless there is a formal system for the identification of training needs. Beishon *et al.* argue that: 'without a formal system of assessment, decisions that are made with regard to promotion ... will be seen as being subjective ... (and) ... such decisions, if not based on objective and clearly stated criteria, may be increasingly viewed as potentially discriminatory by ethnic minority nursing staff' (1995: 74). However, the researchers found that only half of their six case study health employers had introduced a formalised system for appraising nursing staff, and that where it had been introduced, it was not applied across all branches of nursing and midwifery, or across all grades of qualified staff (1995: 73).

## The Impact of 'Racism' Upon Applications for Training in Nursing and Midwifery

'Endemic racism' has allegedly forced some minority ethnic nurses to leave the NHS (Nursing Standard, 1992). Moreover, according to a recent report on nursing shortage published by the King's Fund, 'Attracting young black and minority ethnic nurses into the NHS will only work if the NHS tackles institutional racism' (Meadows, Levenson and Baeza, 2000). It is perhaps not surprising that because of their experiences of discrimination some minority ethnic nurses arguably don't want their daughters to go into the profession (Alibhai, 1988: 26). The demise of the black nurse by the year 2000 was even predicted unless remedial recruitment measures are taken (Pearson, 1987: 26), and, even though this is conjectural, it indicates the depth of feeling on the issue. (Data we present in Chapter 4 of this book indicates that this prediction has not yet come true.) Some of the respondents in the nurse education and training institutions where we carried out our research suggested such a 'deterrent-effect' at work (the selection of the institutions and our lines of enquiry are discussed in detail in Chapter 5). For instance, a lecturer involved in recruitment at the Peverell Institute of Health reported that:

> what is coming over loud and clear is the black ethnic minority students have made an informed judgement not to consider nursing because their mums and dads have not been treated very well as workers, because their aunties, mums and dads have not been treated as patients very well and that does actually become a profession which they don't actually want to dabble into (053).[1]

The Head of the Devonport Institute of Health made a similar point:

> I think a number of Afro-Caribbean community, who did come forward in large numbers into nursing at one stage, have an experience of the enrolled nurse pathway, as distinct from the registered pathway, and you could well have mums and dads feeding the information now onto their children to say 'we got a very raw deal from becoming, by becoming, nurses. We were given this second class approach'. I don't get many second generation Afro-Caribbean people applying to us ... there are more ethnic minority students being deterred from

> working in the NHS by parents and relations who've had previous experience, or dare I say, even current experience, of the NHS. One of the frequent comments passed to me by staff is 'if I had a son or daughter I would not encourage them to work in the NHS and I would not encourage them to be a nurse' (005).

The impact of 'racism' on applications is, however, complex. As we discuss in Chapter 4, applications data show that whilst the discrimination experienced by earlier generations of Black nurses in the NHS may have a deterrent effect on potential Black applicants, it does not appear to be a sufficient deterrent to lead to an under-representation of the groups amongst applicants for training in nursing and midwifery compared with their representation in the population as a whole in England.

In the case of the Asian communities, the picture is also complex. Some commentators have suggested that processes operating within Asian communities, such as cultural norms (Karseras and Hopkins, 1987: 27; Rashid, 1990: 52-3) and career aspirations (Cassidy, 1995), deter young people from the communities concerned from pursuing a career in nursing and midwifery. Such a conclusion had been drawn by a number of respondents in the case study institutions. For instance, the Contracts Manager at the Wembury Institute argued that:

> Although we try to target locally, recruit locally, go to schools and colleges locally, people from the Asian community don't come into nursing and it seems that that is a cultural thing, that ... nursing's not an occupation that's attractive to those groups for cultural reasons ... I think that however hard you tried here to target the local Asian community they still wouldn't come because you can't change the cultural perception of nursing activities for that community ... We've got quite a few Asian women working here, mostly administrators ... and they're from the local community ... it's quite interesting talking to them ... they wouldn't come in as nurses and neither would any of their family because the cultural taboos are just too great ... so you're kind of on a losing wicket really (035).

The view that young people from Asian communities are not interested in nursing as a career also appeared to be supported by some local research in another area. The Administration Manager for the Devonport Institute of Health pointed out that:

> I think for instance (Devonport) has got quite a high proportion of Asian people and that's not reflected in the number of students that we have. When we were part of Devonport College, Devonport Health Authority actually did do a piece of research on that, they engaged somebody to undertake a project and it was quite extensive ... what they came back with was that the perception of nursing was that it wasn't the sort of right status for the people to want to come in to and it was those sort of attitudes that we were up against and there was not a lot that we could do to change that (004).

A lecturer at the Lipson Institute of Health also believed that nursing was regarded as a low status occupation by some minority ethnic communities:

> The Bengali community for example don't perceive nursing to be a, what's the word, good enough, it's too servile ... it was interesting because the open day I talked about ... we had some interesting questions from the Bengali students but there was a reticence there because and you could sense that was why they didn't necessarily want to be in that kind of environment ... they didn't think it would be acceptable to their community (072).

These views were also reflected in institutions which had made very active efforts to recruit applicants from minority ethnic groups. A senior administrator responsible for recruitment in the Mannamead Institute of Health commented:

> I don't want to sound controversial here but I think it's a two-way thing. It's okay opening up and saying 'look we want you to come to us', but they've got to come to us as well. It's okay having policies and open procedures ... but the other end of the scale the families have got, we would like them to allow people to come here (003).

She believed that often young people in the communities concerned were restrained by their parents:

> the lack of interest is not a problem with us, we get people inquiring ... Interest is not a problem, it's people being allowed to come forward and we have people who withdraw at the last minute ... it's getting this over to people that if someone's worked hard to get in please let them start. But we know they have arranged marriages, we know these things happen, and that's what normally happens to us. People get as far as being offered an interview, they don't turn up at interview. They get as far as being offered a place, medical, the lot, then they have to withdraw. I mean our course that started last October, a month before it was due to start four of the students were still in Pakistan and I didn't know whether they were going to be back or not, and they were as it happened, but we lost two others (003).

Similarly, a senior nurse lecturer at the Eggbuckland Institute stated:

> if you were to look say at north ... where you've got quite a high Asian, Bangladeshi population, their parents don't want them to do nursing ... they're all doing pharmacy, dentistry and medicine ... it's not necessarily about the fact we're not recruiting them, it's just they don't want to do nursing (010).

According to a recruitment team leader at the Peveril Institute of Health, this lack of interest did not just apply to Asian communities:

> we were out at a recruitment event here in (Peverell) we had a very nice West Indian couple come with their daughter and you know, we were sort of leaping about and saying can we interest you, you know, and this West Indian lady looked at me and she said 'no thank you honey', she said 'I want better than nursing for my daughter', and our experience, a lot of our experience, particularly with the people from the Caribbean is that they do want better, and certainly as well, people from Asian countries, because their children are often very high achievers (019).

Commentators favouring the 'deterrent-effect' hypothesis discussed above have challenged such assertions about the impact of 'cultural' values. The King's Fund Equal Opportunities Task Force (1990: 11-12) argued that the culture-effect hypothesis is simplistic because it neglects processes operating within health service employment. For instance, the Task Force cited Lee-Cunin's (1989) finding that among young Asian women respondents, twice as many suggested that 'racism' and discrimination were disincentives to a career in nursing and midwifery, as those who suggested that their families would not approve of such a career choice. In the context of such findings Ward (1993) argued that the culture-effect hypothesis fails 'to acknowledge that the views people have of a service or institution, in this case the National Health Service, are not merely a product of cultural beliefs but also their experiences of and within those institutions' (1993: 172).

Neither the 'deterrent-effect' hypothesis, nor the 'culture-effect' hypothesis, exclusive of the other, adequately accounts for the patterns of application from Britain's minority ethnic communities for training in the health professions. This is clearly evident in the case of minority ethnic applicants to medical school who are 'over-represented' despite the long history of disadvantage and discrimination experienced by overseas and minority ethnic doctors. In providing a perspective on how career choices are made, Esmail has suggested that 'there are often wider social and cultural reasons why, in some higher education institutions, the student body does not reflect the proportionality in terms of gender and ethnicity of the wider society. The high proportion of Asian students in medicine is almost certainly a reflection of the fact that a large number of Asian doctors work in the NHS as a result of immigration policies that encouraged Asian doctors to come and work in the NHS in the 1960s and 1970s ... As with white students in medicine, choice of profession partly reflects the views of parents ...' (Esmail, 2001: 82). In contrast, in the case of the nursing and midwifery professions, from the anecdotal evidence discussed in this chapter, past experience of discrimination and disadvantage appears to be a plausible deterrent, when combined with other aspects of choice, affecting potential applicants from minority ethnic communities. In Chapter 3 we examine how the NHS has responded to the evidence of racial discrimination and disadvantage at work, and in the rest of the book we examine applications to nursing and midwifery training, and the recruitment and selection processes involved.

## Note

1 Respondent number.

# 3 Equal Opportunity Policy and the NHS

How has the NHS responded to the discrimination and disadvantage experienced by health service workers from minority ethnic communities? Arguably, over the last 25 years, there have been significant achievements in the development and implementation of equal opportunity policies in the health services. However, up until the early 1980s the Department of Health failed to provide an immonstrable lead to the NHS on equal opportunity policy. That failure was due in part to the prevailing management style that was more 'administrative' than 'managerial'. There was also a prevailing view that the substantial numbers of black and minority ethnic workers employed in the health services indicated the absence of a problem of discrimination. Two decades later there was considerable policy exhortation, from the centre, for the implementation of equal opportunity policies in the NHS. This chapter evaluates the factors that have steered this course of policy development.

We observe that policy initiatives have been shaped by a combination of pressure from outside the health services, and the innovation and commitment of some individuals strategically placed within the NHS. Most of all, however, pragmatism has arguably been the driving force. To indicate how arguments for policy implementation have increasingly been framed in terms of self-interest, or a 'business-case', we focus on the emergence of such policy exhortation until it was fully articulated in the early 1990s. Our evaluation of the policy process draws from discussions with health service equal opportunity specialists, senior civil servants, and health service managers, carried out in 1991 and 1992.[1] Gergen (1968: 207) has recommended that one of the more productive means of studying the process of public policy formation is to concentrate on individuals who exercise considerable 'leverage' or power in the shaping of policy. Accordingly, most of the respondents were key actors involved in the policy process at national level for the NHS. There were a few respondents who were only marginally involved in the national policy process, but their role afforded them with a view of the policy process overall. Some had made a considerable impact on the policy process through their research and publications. Lengthy discussions were held with eighteen key informants in total. Each informant was guaranteed anonymity, so we are not able to name them. Informants were identified through a 'snowballing process', following an initial approach to the King's Fund Equal Opportunities Task Force.

Each informant was asked to provide their own interpretation of the process of development of equal opportunity policy at national level for the NHS. They were also asked to identify what factors they thought were influential for policy development; and to account for the role of their institution and their own role in the policy process. As a check on the validity of their interpretations each informant was asked to indicate how their role provided them with an informed view of the policy process rather than it being merely conjectural. Throughout, the research involved an inductive process involving 'detective work', 'following one lead to another' and looking for 'patterns' and 'consistencies' in the data (Mintzberg, 1983: 108). Whilst the research initially began without any prior hypotheses, preliminary hypotheses were formulated from the very first interview and they provided part of the topic guide for subsequent interviews. In essence then, the analysis began with the first piece of data collected. Care was taken, however, to avoid premature closure of avenues of enquiry by continuing to investigate avenues that did not accord with the emerging hypotheses.

## 'Hands-off' Managerial Style

The first significant activity on equal opportunities at national-level for the NHS was the issuing of a circular (U.K. Department of Health and Social Security, 1978) to Health Authorities and Boards of Governors following the 1976 Race Relations Act. The London Association of Community Relations Councils (LACRC) described the circular as 'one of the few positive and imaginative responses made by Government to the passing of the Race Relations Act' (LACRC, 1985: 8). The circular contained a number of recommendations for policy implementation. Health Authorities were advised to review their recruitment criteria, and job specifications in particular, to ensure that they do not have the potential for indirect discrimination. They were also advised to review their practices concerning the selection, training, promotion and transfer of staff, to ensure that they are free from direct and potential indirect discrimination. Authorities were advised to attempt to achieve more than just bare compliance with the Race Relations Act. It was recommended that:

> employment policies and practices should therefore include effective procedures to ensure equality of opportunity for members of minority groups. This can best be achieved by developing a policy which is clearly stated, known to all employees, and has and is seen to have the backing of senior management, is effectively supervised, provides a periodic feedback of information to senior management, and is seen to work in practice (U.K. Department of Health and Social Security 1978, para. 14).

The circular also drew attention to the provisions of the 1976 Race Relations Act concerning the exceptions for genuine occupational qualifications (1976 Race Relations Act: section 5) (U.K. Department of Health and Social Security, 1978, para. 15) and to the positive action provisions of the Act (1976 Race Relations Act: sections 37 and 38).

With the benefit of hindsight, the recommendations were very innovative, as over two decades later they now constitute core equal opportunity measures adopted by many employers. But at the time the circular arguably had little impact on policy implementation on the ground. One senior manager (102) interviewed said that in the Health Authority where she worked the circular was simply 'filed away' and forgotten about. This shouldn't be surprising as historically the recommendations contained in circulars issued by the centre have been for policy guidance, and not mandatory. Because they lack teeth, the issuing of circulars has generally been regarded as an ineffective means of developing policy (Brown, 1962: 371-74; Stewart and Sleeman, 1967, Ham, 1981: 184; Klein, 1983: 51; McNaught, 1988: 71).

The London Association of Community Relations Councils argued in their 1985 report *In a Critical Condition* - that some of the responsibility for the lack of action on the part of Health Authorities in response to the circular rested back at the centre with the Department of Health and Social Security. According to the LACRC, the DHSS:

> appears to have done nothing to follow up the circular; it has never asked authorities to what extent they have acted on the advice given, and it has never issued any further advice on equal opportunities. (LACRC, 1985: 8).

The lack of action at the time by the DHSS was also raised by the House of Commons Home Affairs Committee in 1981. It is instructive to read the exchange on this question between the committee chairman and the Under Secretary for Social Services - Mr. Scott Whyte:

> (Chairman) So far as promotion of equal opportunities is concerned, back in October 1978 following the 1976 Race Relations Act, the Department issued guidance to the Health Authorities and others, I think, urging the need for positive equal opportunities policies. Has there been any follow up to that? Have you monitored the extent to which Area Health Authorities and others have been pursuing those equal employment policies?
>
> (Mr. Scott Whyte) No, we have not done this, partly because the extent of our monitoring the activities of both health and local authorities is something which we have been reducing, but also because those policies laid down in the Race Relations Act were really full legal obligations on employing authorities. They were not policies being recommended to them by the Government. The Act, of course, contains its own system of enforcement of the obligations which does not involve any participation by the Secretary of State so there is not really a case - it would seem a work of supererogation - for us to monitor the extent to which authorities are conforming with the law.
>
> (Chairman) It is not clear to me why you issue guidance, if that is the case, but you do.
>
> (Mr. Scott Whyte) It is normal practice to draw the attention of health and local authorities to any changes in the law which affect their operations. At the time when an Act is passed or regulations are made, we draw the local authorities' attention to this new feature of the

> landscape that they have got to work in (U.K. House of Commons, 1981: 195).

Even if the circular was simply drawing the attention of Health Authorities to the requirements of the Race Relations Act - and it arguably went much further than that in the recommendations it made - why did the Department not take a more active role in policy implementation? One answer seems to be that it did not regard discrimination as a serious problem in the NHS. This was clearly the Department's view in the mid-1970s. In its submission to the 1975 Select Committee on Race Relations and Immigration it stated that:

> Although the Department is not complaisant, the policy that all eligible persons shall have equal opportunities for employment and advancement would seem to be working adequately in the NHS, if measured by the low volume of complaints ... It is, we feel, universally recognised that the NHS would have had the most serious staffing difficulties many years ago at all levels and in all professions if it had not an employment policy towards staff that disregarded race, colour, ethnic or national origins (U.K. House of Commons, 1975: 191).

The Department's recognition of discrimination at work in the NHS might have begun to evolve shortly after it provided the above submission to the Select Committee, as in 1976 in the *Quarterly Journal of the Employment Section of the Community Relations Commission* it was observed that:

> Black workers, irrespective of occupational status, find their job experience in the NHS structured by institutional racialism - this is the over-view which we gain when the fragments of information are pieced together. Remarkably, it is acquiring a consensual position among the administrative elites (in the DHSS, the GMS, the medical schools ...). The real debate begins when we ask: what is to be done? (Grainger, 1976: 12).

If a consensual position had indeed emerged, it was not followed up by any action - apart from issuing the circular. This was despite indications of discrimination against overseas doctors produced by the Policy Studies

Institute in 1980 (Smith, 1980). The inactivity of the Department was summed up by the House of Commons Home Affairs Committee in 1981:

> The Department of Health and Social Security apparently have neither Minister nor staff with a particular responsibility for combating racial disadvantage ... . There is little or no evidence that the Department are aware of the implications for their areas of responsibility of the wide range of racial disadvantage. Local authority social services departments and local Health Authorities are perforce aware of such matters and have taken a variety of administrative steps towards dealing with them. The department have not, and would not appear to have taken the lead in advising authorities on good policy and practice (U.K. House of Commons, 1981: xxi).

Despite the Select Committee's belief that local Health Authorities had taken 'a variety of administrative steps' to combat racial disadvantage the LACRC research on the implementation of equal employment opportunities policies, indicates on the contrary - in the case of London - that such action had only been taken by a few Health Authorities.

The failure of the Department to take the lead on policy implementation needs to be considered in the context of the prevailing management style in the NHS in the late 1970s and early 1980s. This was characterised - by one official interviewed - as a 'hands-off' approach between management at the centre and local management in Health Authorities:

> the 1978 circular ... was simply telling Authorities what was in the Race Relations Act and advising them as to how they should deal with it, and that was the style then. We launched our guidance on the waters and watched with interest to see what happened to it, but we didn't actively pursue it ... and it was only really post the Griffiths Report with the establishment of the Management Board that we got into the style of pursuing things with a formal review process to do it in.
>
> In the early 1980s it was always a very much hands-off approach. In the early years of the (Conservative) Government, it was cut down the Civil Service, reduce the functions, get as much out of the Department as

> much as you can, and there was no sense in which the Management Executive were managing the health service ... (104).

In the early 1980s riots occurred in urban areas with significant concentrations of minority ethnic communities. They produced a variety of social policy responses (Young, 1983). For the NHS - at local level - in areas where riots occurred, there also appeared to be some policy impact. McNaught, for instance, observed in his study of West Lambeth Health Authority that the Brixton riots added a greater impetus to emergent policies concerning both equal employment opportunities and services sensitive to the needs of minority ethnic groups (McNaught, 1988: 115-6). The publication of the Scarman Report (U.K. Home Office, 1981) appears to have been influential in the decision of the West Lambeth District Management Team in 1982 to proceed with an audit of the ethnic composition of the workforce proposed by the District Personnel Officer. This reversed an earlier rejection of the proposal (McNaught 1988: 93), but the impact of the riots upon the Department of Heath, and consequently the development of equal opportunity policy across the NHS, appears to have been limited.

## Developing Equal Opportunity Policy Expertise

The publication in 1984 of the Commission for Racial Equality's *Code of Practice* (CRE, 1984a) - containing recommendations for the implementation of equal opportunity policies - marked the beginning of a new phase in the policy process. There was a considerable increase in policy activity compared to the earlier lack of action. The CRE followed up publication its *Code* with an approach to the Department of Health. According to one official interviewed:

> the CRE approached us at that time and said 'isn't it about time you updated your circular?' (104).

The publication of the *Code of Practice* and the approach by the CRE occurred in the context of a change in management style in the NHS that meant that the Department would take a more directive role:

> We'd just got the Griffiths Report - which was in October 1983 - and we were beginning to consider how to re-build the system so that the centre was managerial rather than administrative, if I can use that over-simplifying distinction. We didn't actually go much on issuing circulars, and we thought then that what was needed was some kind of body which would help to drive the thing (104).

Officials interviewed concurred that the need for a 'body' to lead policy development was justified by the Department of Health on the grounds of a lack of appropriate expertise within the health service:

> this was a subject on which frankly very little had been done other than to try and protect ... other than Authorities trying to protect themselves from legal action ... and not always successfully at that, and there was very little expertise out there. So the first task that was set to was to make it easier for them. If we'd said to every Authority 'Prepare an equal opportunities policy' they'd have to start from scratch ... somebody in a personnel department somewhere was familiar with the legislation and could advise people on it ... but there weren't people out there who had written policies ... or very few of them ... or had any experience of developing and running a pro-active policy (104).

The Department's perceived need to establish a body of expertise coincided with an emerging interest in equal opportunities by the King Edward's Hospital Fund for London (King's Fund). The eventual outcome - after approximately eighteen months of negotiations - was the establishment of an Equal Opportunities Task Force in May 1986 under the auspices of the King's Fund. One senior manager described the convergence of interests:

> They (the Department of Health) felt that it wasn't appropriate to have a unit within the Department. That what was appropriate was a unit placed somewhere outside, and the King's Fund was the obvious institution to approach to ask to take on a Task Force, so they approached the King's Fund. This tied in with ... ideas which the Chief Executive of the King's Fund had at the time that he would like to extend what the King's Fund was doing in the equal opportunities field (101).

It appears, however, that the CRE - which originally stimulated the activity by the Department - had reservations about the establishment of the Task Force:

> their reservations were that they felt that the initiative that was required was for the Department nationally to in some way direct Health Authorities to implement the Code of Practice. I think what they were suggesting was another circular to Health Authorities, which at the time the CRE felt would be the answer (101).

Despite the CRE's apparent reservations, however, they subsequently accepted representation on the membership of the Task Force. In addition to the CRE's pressure on the Department, the Equal Opportunities Commission also began to apply some pressure:

> So we launched the Task Force, then there was a certain amount of disquiet around from the Equal Opportunities Commission and from (within the Department) that we weren't addressing equal opportunity issues for women (104).

It was decided that two organisations should be established to develop the expertise for equal employment-opportunities policy separately on the basis of 'race' and sex. In negotiations between the Department of Health and the King's Fund:

> the case was argued there for looking at equal opportunities in employment right across the board. One of the reasons that we decided against that was because it would have left out the service link for ethnic minorities. But another strong reason is that any single body looking at that whole area which is in any way representative becomes gigantic and very readily descends into a 'talk shop'. The way to overcome that is to appoint a small group of individuals for their expertise (104).

A key reason behind the establishment of separate organisations appears to have been a desire to establish the 'confidence' of representatives from minority ethnic groups:

> The problem that we had there was that we couldn't have people readily available from within the health service or close to the health service who would actually have the confidence of all the groups, and a good deal of the purpose of the Task Force and the National Steering Group has been to build confidence. And we felt that it was necessary if the ethnic minorities themselves were to believe that what was being done was seriously directed towards their interests to have a body which had a substantial ethnic minority membership on it, and which was, as it were, dedicated to their interests. They would have suspected if we'd set up a body to look right across the board that it would focus primarily on gender issues (104).

Therefore, in addition to the King's Fund Equal Opportunities Task Force, the National Steering Group for Women was established in December 1986. Both organisations produced written policy guidance that was disseminated to Health Authorities. One major aim of the Task Force was to:

> try to encourage role models - to help those Authorities that were most advanced to continue to advance, so that their examples could be used by other Health Authorities. (The Task Force) also tried to help equal opportunities advisers, because it has seen that as one other way that equal opportunities development was going to come about (101).

The introduction of equal opportunities into the NHS annual review process in 1988 marked a new development in the policy process. The annual Ministerial review of Health Regions - and in turn the review of Districts by Regions - was established in 1982 (Allsop, 1984; Levitt and Wall, 1984). The review was strengthened by the introduction of a system of performance reviews of Regions by the NHS Management Board (now called the NHS Management Executive) in 1986 (Mills, 1987). The strengthened annual review process provided a potential mechanism to hold Regions, and in turn Districts, accountable for equal opportunity policy implementation.

By 1988, sufficient equal opportunity expertise appears to have been generated for the NHS for policy implementation to be included in the review process:

> The timing was calculated in relation to the progress which the Task Force and the National Steering Group had made ... 1988 was the right timing in terms of there being enough material now available for Authorities being able to pick that up and turn it into working policies relatively painlessly ... there were a number of Districts who had made progress from whom you could network and there was varying levels of interest and expertise in regions, and more so in Districts - and that's still the case - but there were enough people ready to go, and there was enough material ready for them to build on (104).

Two further, but opposing, factors also occurred in the late 1980s and early 1990s. In 1991 re-organisation of the NHS devolved accountability away from the centre - the Department of Health - to health service employers. The re-organisation was a weakening of the influence of the centre on policy implementation. The opposing process involved a growing recognition of a potential labour shortage facing the NHS. That recognition provided a significant stimulus for policy implementation.

## Policy Pragmatism

The equal opportunities policy process for the NHS in the late 1980s and early 1990s was characterised by a consensus amongst the key players in relation to the stimulus for policy implementation. The consensus was remarkable as some of the organisations involved brought competing interests to the policy process. In addition to the Department of Health, groups established to develop equal opportunities expertise for the NHS - the National Steering Group for Women in the NHS and the King's Fund Equal Opportunities Task Force - the Equal Opportunities Commission, the training arm of the NHS Management Executive - the NHS Training Authority (latterly the NHS Training Directorate) - and the trades unions all argued that the implementation of equal employment-opportunities policies by Health Authorities was essential - in the context of a labour supply crisis - to retain existing staff and attract additional sources of workers. In addition, the recruitment of health service workers from minority ethnic communities was promoted on the grounds of improving the quality of services to the communities concerned. We discuss both of these pragmatic policy imperatives in turn below.

*The Demographic 'Time-Bomb'*

In the late 1980s there was a growing realisation that the NHS, and the nursing profession in particular, was facing a 'demographic time-bomb' (cf. U.K. Employment Department, 1988). As a result of a decline in the birth-rate in the 1960s and 1970s there had been a fall since the early 1980s in the number of young people in the labour market, whilst the population as a whole continued to grow. As the NHS had traditionally recruited a substantial number of school-leavers it had been facing a growing shortage of labour. In the case of nurses, constituting approximately half of the NHS labour force, new recruits had normally been drawn from school-leavers, primarily women. However, this potential pool of labour had been declining. For instance, between 1982 - when there was a peak in the supply of sixteen to nineteen year-olds (3,712,000) - and the trough in supply in 1994 (2,602,000), the number of both male and female sixteen to nineteen year-olds fell by approximately 30 per cent (U.K. Employment Department, 1992: 176-77). The number of female school-leavers with between five 'O' Levels and two 'A' Levels - the traditional pool of recruitment for nursing students - declined to a lesser extent during this period (22 per cent between 1983 and 1993) but the difference was eroded by an increasing number entering further and higher education (Conroy and Stidston, 1988: 5).

The fall in the supply of potential labour was matched during the 1980s by a fall in the annual number of trainee nurses. The number of student nurses declined from their peak in 1984 (54,418) to a low in 1987 (50,875), and then began to rise again. The rise was primarily due to the increasing number of male student nurses whose total increased by nearly 33 per cent between 1984 and 1989 (5,646 to 7,487) whilst the number of female student nurses declined by 7 per cent during the same period (48,772 to 45,354). The number of trainee nurses overall though - when taking the lower training grade of pupil nurse into account - fell considerably during the 1980s. The number of pupil nurses fell by 80 per cent between 1981 and 1989 (21,254 to 4,179) as a consequence of the phasing out of two-tier nurse training. The rise in the number of student nurses in the late 1980s did not compensate for the decline in the number of pupil nurses, and there was a consistent annual fall between 1982 and 1989 in the total number of trainee nurses, falling by 24 per cent in total (75,402 to 57,020) (U.K. Department of Health and Social Security, 1987: table 3.17, p.54; U.K. Department of Health, 1991a: table 3.18, p.54).

The decline in the supply of potential new recruits to the nursing labour force coincided with a growing demand for NHS services. At the same time, the potential staffing crisis facing the NHS was amplified, during the period in question, by growing competition from the service sector for the same pool of female labour. In the context of a diminished supply of labour in general for the nursing workforce, the potential labour supply from Britain's minority ethnic communities had been growing in significance. This is because the age profile of each of the black and Asian minority ethnic groups is younger in comparison with the population as a whole. They thus represent a significant pool of potential young workers. For instance, in the 1991 population Census one-third of the ethnic minorities as a whole were aged under sixteen years compared with nearly one-fifth (19 per cent) of the white population. Similarly, whilst the minority ethnic groups accounted for 5.5 per cent of the population overall, they accounted for nearly twice this proportion (9.0 per cent) of under sixteen year-olds (U.K. Office of Population Censuses and Surveys, 1993).

The significance of the minority ethnic communities as a source of labour for the NHS was clearly recognised in health policy circles. For instance, on the launch of a 'Management Guide' to the implementation of equal employment-opportunities policies in the NHS (NHS Training Authority, 1989) the Minister of Health warned health service employers who failed to provide equality of opportunity for women and minority ethnic staff that they faced a 'staffing crisis of unprecedented proportions' (U.K. Department of Health, 1989). He stated that:

> Equal opportunities is not just about social justice - important though that is. As every good employer well knows, equal opportunities has a more practical dimension, namely securing a future workforce in terms of numbers and quality and making the best use of our most valuable resource - our staff ... As a labour-intensive organisation, the looming shortage of staff - especially skilled - must surely be one of the greatest challenges confronting the NHS over the next decade ... equal

> opportunity must be addressed as part of mainstream management practice to ensure the NHS attracts and keeps the staff it needs to meet the demand placed upon it ... Unless that is done quickly the service could find itself confronting a staffing crisis of unprecedented proportions. That is why in the short time still available managers must give this matter their full and urgent attention (U.K. Department of Health, 1989).

Nearly three years later, the then Minister for Health - Virginia Bottomley - stated publicly in promoting the equal opportunities initiatives of the 'Opportunity 2000' campaign in the NHS that it was 'not a philanthropic exercise ... but enlightened self-interest' (Iganski, 1993a). The Department of Health launched a number of major equal employment-opportunities initiatives for women in the NHS in 1991 and 1992, and they were promoted primarily both on the grounds of recruitment and retention of female labour, and an efficiency argument concerning the most cost-effective use of labour. For instance, at the launch of the 'Women in the NHS' initiative in June 1991 (U.K. Department of Health, 1991b) Virginia Bottomley argued that:

> The NHS employs more people and more women in particular than any other organisation in Europe. As demographic changes intensify competition for the best school-leavers, the NHS must be in the forefront. It must become a by-word for good 'women friendly' employment practices (U.K. Department of Health, 1991c).

Similarly, in October - shortly before the establishment of the NHS 'Women's Unit' in November 1991 (U.K. Department of Health, 1991d) - the Health Minister again argued that:

> Equal opportunities is not just about social justice - important though that is. As every good employer knows, equal opportunities has a more practical dimension. It is about securing the right number of qualified staff to meet future needs. It is about making the best possible use of our most valuable resource - our workforce (U.K. Department of Health, 1991e).

The contribution made by equal employment-opportunities policies to the efficient use of human resources was emphasised by Duncan Nichol - the Chief Executive of the NHS - in the NHS Management Executive's 'Good Practice Handbook' for 'Women in the NHS', launched in October 1991 (U.K. Department of Health, 1991e), who stated that:

> The NHS employs more than a million people. Over 75 per cent of these are women. Managers have a clear business responsibility to ensure that they make the best possible use of these valuable people. The health service simply cannot afford to lose these skilled and expensively trained staff. It ought to be leading the way in implementing employment and career progression policies which are not only compatible with the particular needs of women staff, but which also make sound business sense. This is a necessity if we are to continue to recruit and retain the services of good quality staff. That is why we at the centre are committed to a policy of improving opportunities for women across all disciplines and at all levels (U.K. NHS Management Executive, 1991).

Similar arguments for broadening recruitment were reiterated in the late 1980s and early 1990s by the King's Fund Equal Opportunities Task Force, the NHS Training Directorate and the health service trades unions (Iganski, 1993b: 191-192). The apparent value of an equal opportunity policy in relation to the recruitment, retention, and the most efficient use of labour, has also been a prominent argument behind policy exhortation from the NHS staff-side organisations. For example, the National Union of Public Employees (NUPE) in its submissions to the Nursing Staff, Midwives and Health Visitors Pay Review Body (cf. NUPE, 1989; 1990), as well as emphasising the importance of pay to the recruitment and retention of staff, argued in the case of women workers that:

> the NHS must attract experienced nursing staff back to the service and recruit women returning to work after bringing up children. But competition for women, particularly women returners, will grow fiercer through the 1990s, as industry and commerce also look to recruit from these labour sources. Those employers who can offer women career development opportunities, and a flexible pattern of work to fit in with

> their domestic commitments, will be the most successful in the competition for employees (NUPE, 1990: 3-4).

In the case of black minority ethnic nurses NUPE also argued that:

> The NHS will also need to tap into non-traditional recruitment markets. This means reversing the growing shortage of black and ethnic minority nurses, by checking their departure from the NHS, attracting back those who have left, and encouraging more young black people into nursing (NUPE, 1990: 4).

A focus on the labour and skills shortage was also significantly at the centre of the Equal Opportunities Commission's strategic plan for the 1990s, and their strategy of intervention in the NHS in particular. In specifying their strategy for the 1990s the Commission hailed a new era in their approach to equal opportunities. It planned a shift in strategy from moral exhortation for policy implementation to a more persuasive approach by profiling the potential contribution of women in the labour market in the context of the projected shortage of young workers. In their strategy document *From Policy to Practice* the Commission announced:

> Our strategy focuses more directly and with greater priority on the task of making fully available to society the skills which women can provide. We shall change from being an organisation largely engaged in securing equal rights for women into a body which can also play a major role in achieving central national economic objectives through the implementation of effective equal opportunities practice (EOC, 1988).

The tenor of the Commission's strategy document was that the 'demographic time-bomb' provided the most expeditious moment for persuading employers and policy-makers to establish equal opportunities practices and improve the material position of women in the labour market. The new strategy of the Equal Opportunities Commission for the 1990s coincided from 1990 with the Commission's strategic focus on the NHS. That focus was part of a continuing strategy of concentrating their efforts on one distinct area of employment after another and, prior to the NHS, employment in police forces in Britain had been targeted for attention. The interest in the NHS appeared to have emerged (in addition to the obvious consequences of the demographic timebomb because the NHS is such a large employer of women) from the involvement of the Chair of the EOC in 1988 - Baroness Platt of Writtle - in meetings with senior health service managers via the Royal Institute of Public Administration where she learnt about the slow progress of equal opportunities policy implementation in the NHS. Although there was no regular formal liaison between the EOC and the Department of Health, Baroness Platt subsequently approached the then Health Minister, Barney Hayhoe, to push for top level commitment to policy implementation by the Department. There was some surprise in the Commission at the apparent 'hands-off' approach to equal opportunities in Health Authorities by the Department of Health, and according to the EOC's Director of Development Patrick Walker - in his speech at a King's Fund seminar in May 1990 - the Commission was attempting to take a 'strong line' with Ministers with the 'intention to keep up pressure from the top downwards on the whole issue of equal opportunities.' In keeping with the EOC's strategy for the 1990s their approach to the NHS was to focus on the potential labour and skills shortage and the consequent contribution that could be made by women. One influential aspect of the EOC's focus on the NHS was a survey and subsequent report published in August 1991 of the extent of equal employment-opportunities policy implementation by Health Authorities across the NHS, which demonstrated that the NHS as a whole had still much to achieve (EOC, 1991). According to one respondent from the Department of Health (108) the Department wanted to be seen to 'do something' before the survey findings were made public. The Personnel Directorate of the NHS Management Executive consequently commissioned the Office for Public Management to produce a report which detailed the experience of women workers in the NHS, initiatives taken, and a strategy to improve the position of women overall (Goss and Brown, 1991).

Overall, it was a deliberate strategy on the part of the Equal Opportunities Commission to promote policy by using a language that health service managers would both understand and listen to. The strategy was a response to the feedback from some health service managers to the EOC that the commitment of managers in general was more likely to be secured by a 'business' argument - by appealing to their 'pragmatic instincts' (105) - rather than a moral argument. In this context, the demographic 'time-bomb' provided - in the words of one official (107) interviewed - a 'sweet gift' to the

EOC. As Patrick Walker - the EOC's Director of Development at the time - stated at a King's Fund seminar in May 1990:

> People tell us one way of getting through to managers is to talk about skill shortages, but as far as we are concerned we are talking about equal opportunities.

This would seem to be a perfectly rational and effective strategy, as what better time - an official (102) in the Department of Health asked - to push for equal opportunity policy when there is a labour shortage? Likewise another official in the Department reported that:

> The moral issue is still rather a minority support amongst health service people, but there is a strong recognition - and quite a lot of people probably wouldn't be giving the thing priority on moral grounds - that we do need to tackle it on recruitment, retention, and best use of skills grounds ... So we began with a social approach to it if you like, and that's gradually moved over time to there being a very strong recruitment, retention etc, basis to it, and frankly that's getting more done than any amount of preaching (104).

The need for this deliberate pragmatic strategy had already been recognised by the National Steering Group for Women in the NHS in the late 1980s. In introducing its guide to the implementation of equal opportunity policies in the NHS, the Chair of the Steering Group - Victor Flintham - reported that:

> The Group started work in earnest in 1986 and from the beginning adopted a pragmatic, rather than a philosophical, approach to its work. It seemed to us that appeals for positive action from the NHS management would only succeed if we focused on managerial needs and concerns (National Steering Group for Women in the NHS, 1989: 1).

Likewise, in the preface to the 'Management Guide' to the implementation of equal opportunity policy, the Chair of the NHS Training Authority made it clear that:

> Equal opportunities is thus much more than natural justice, it is a practical imperative to assist managers in resolving staffing issues and improving service delivery (NHS Training Authority, 1989: 3).

*Health Services Sensitive to Minority Ethnic Communities*

A large body of literature and research evidence has now accumulated revealing inadequacies in health care provision for Britain's black and Asian minority ethnic communities. The literature has been reviewed elsewhere (McNaught, 1988; Kushnick, 1988; Smaje, 1995; Mason, 2000). But it is useful to discuss it briefly here because the inadequacies have been used as a significant justification - in policy exhortation - for equal opportunity policy for employment in the NHS. Brent Community Health Council published one of the earliest critical accounts of service delivery in 1981. Their report argued that the culture and specific needs of black people had neither been acknowledged nor catered for by the NHS. Controversially, the report also argued that the NHS was involved in the State's alleged efforts to control the number of black people in Britain by promoting contraception, including the controversial contraceptive injection *Depo-Provera*. The report alleged that 'More leaflets have been produced in Asian languages on birth control than any other topic', and some women from minority ethnic groups reportedly felt that they had been offered abortions and sterilisations more readily and more frequently than white women (Brent CHC, 1981: 21-22).

The Black Health Workers and Patients Group also controversially argued in 1983 that 'black cultures' have been regarded as pathological by some health professionals (Black Health Workers and Patients Group, 1983: 54). In the case of mental health services other critics alleged that the role of racism in the aetiology of mental illness was little understood (Burke, 1984: 1, Health and Race 1986: 1). McNaught (1984: 24-27; 1988: 58-59) presented a synopsis of additional alleged 'discrimination' faced by black people at the hands of health service professionals. In relation to nursing care, for instance, it was alleged that black patients had been treated in an 'offhand' manner; subjected to derogatory comments; and administered unnecessary medication. The National Association for Health Authorities in 1988 argued that overall few Health Authorities had provision for the needs of minority ethnic groups in their planning and delivery of service (National Association of Health Authorities, 1988: 8).

The more recent literature indicates that the early criticisms are still pertinent. Language and cultural differences between health care professionals and users of services have continued to inhibit access to health services by some minority ethnic groups in, for example, general practice (Mehta, 1993; Leisten and Richardson, 1996; Nazroo, 1997), mental health (Au, 1990; CRE, 1991: 8-9; Joyram, 1994), maternity care (Bowler, 1993), and ambulance services (Eaton, 1997). Misdiagnosis and inadequate treatment has also allegedly occurred in the context of cultural misunderstandings between providers and users of services, especially in the case of mental health services (Joyram, 1994). The professional training of health care workers has also arguably been permeated by negative representations and stereotyping of minority ethnic groups (Bowler, 1993; Bhopal and White, 1993), and they have generally been ill-prepared for working in multi-cultural settings (Gerrish *et al.*, 1996). Negative encounters between some minority ethnic users of health services and health care professionals have continued (Bothamley, 1996).

In the context of the inadequacies in health care provision the need to employ health workers from minority ethnic communities - to increase the sensitivity of services to those communities - has been increasingly recognised in health policy circles and by NHS management. It has been used in policy exhortation from the centre as justifying the need for equal opportunity policy - although health services have allegedly lagged behind the personal social services in recognising the value of a diverse workforce (Johnson, 1987; Mehta, 1993).

Barriers to communication - both linguistic and cultural - between members of Asian communities and health service workers were highlighted in the early 1980s during the *Stop Rickets Campaign* funded by the Department of Health and Social Security and targeted on the Asian communities in Britain. The aim of the campaign was to reduce the incidence of rickets amongst those communities through a health education programme aimed at increasing the intake of vitamin D. It was apparent to campaign workers that many individuals in the communities concerned lacked a clear understanding of the extent of NHS services available to them, and similarly the work of many health service professionals was hindered by their lack of understanding of Asian cultures. It was recognised that the employment of health workers with appropriate language skills would improve the delivery and access to health care and it was recommended - in the campaign report -

that effort should be made to increase the numbers of health visitors, school nurses and midwives who could speak Asian languages (Save the Children Fund, 1983: 14-19). The recruitment of health workers from the Asian communities was a central element of a further campaign - the *Asian Mother and Baby Campaign* - organised and funded by the Department of Health and Social Security in the mid 1980s. The origins of that campaign lay in the apparent gap between need and service provision indicated by the earlier *Stop Rickets Campaign.* The *Asian Mother and Baby Campaign* recognised that 'racial stereotyping' by health service professionals in addition to cultural and language differences between potential user and service provider resulted not only in inappropriate service provision, but also discouraged the use of services (U.K. Department of Health and Social Security, 1987b: 12). The employment of eighty 'link-workers' initially funded for two years by the Department of Health and Social Security as part of the campaign was intended to improve communication and understanding between Health Authorities and Asian communities thereby improving the health care of those communities.

In addition to the employment of specialist workers, it was proposed by politicians leading the Department of Health - and others with policy-making influence - that the implementation of equal employment opportunities in general will lead to improved and more sensitive provision of health services to black minority ethnic communities. For instance, in opening a 'Management Seminar' on 'Ethnic Minority Health' in 1987 organised by the Department of Health and Social Security, the Minister for Health - Tony Newton - after stating the Government's commitment to equal employment-opportunities in the NHS, claimed that:

> We are committed as deeply to equal opportunities in service delivery. The two are obviously closely linked. No one would wish to move to a situation where patients were treated only by staff of their own ethnic group. But an NHS which has developed an equal opportunities policy in employment is likely to be - and to be seen to be - more ready to promote equal access to services. And an NHS where there is a better ethnic mix across the hierarchy will be better equipped to identify and remove obstacles to equal access (U.K. Department of Health and Social Security 1988: 2).

Similarly, in introducing its 'model' equal opportunity policy the King's Fund Equal Opportunities Task Force asserted that:

> We believe that by ensuring equal opportunities in employment for ethnic minorities, authorities will be better placed to improve the delivery of service to minority racial groups. We believe also that the health service must benefit from using to the full all the potential talent and experience available from the whole community (KFEOTF, 1987: 3).

The National Association of Health Authorities in its 1988 publication *Action Not Words* also clearly drew the connection between equal opportunity in employment and improvements in health-care delivery by arguing that:

> real improvements in service provision for black and minority ethnic groups in the NHS can only be successful if parallel measures are taken on equal opportunities in employment.
>
> An effective way of making health services responsive to the needs of a multi-racial and multi-cultural population is to ensure that members of minority ethnic groups are employed at all levels in the health service and thus involved automatically in the planning, management and delivery of those services (National Association of Health Authorities, 1988: 10).

More recently, the primary objective of the NHS programme of action on equal opportunity for minority ethnic staff – launched in December 1993 – was to achieve: 'The equitable representation of minority ethnic groups at all levels in the NHS … reflecting the ethnic composition of the local population' on the principle that 'Under-representation of certain ethnic groups in the workforce may affect the ability of a provider to offer services to patients from those groups' (Equal Opportunities Review, 1994: 25-28).

In short, an additional - and prominent - utility argument was used during the late 1980s to justify the implementation of equal opportunity policies in the NHS. The implementation of equal opportunity policies was regarded as a significant measure for the recruitment of black minority ethnic health workers, with consequent improvements to health service delivery to black minority ethnic communities.

## Enlightened Self-interest

Significant advances have been made in the implementation of equal opportunity policies in the NHS since the DHSS issued its circular in 1978 outlining the implications of the 1976 Race Relations Act for NHS. The course of policy development and implementation has been shaped by a combination of pressure from outside the NHS, innovation and commitment of some individuals strategically placed within the NHS, and pragmatic interest. Most of all, though, pragmatism has arguably been the driving force. There was a consensus amongst officials and health service managers interviewed that considerations of justice have played little part in the course of policy development. Rather than using appeals to justice, policy exhortation has appealed to 'good business sense', particularly with regard to the recruitment and retention of health service workers. One senior personnel specialist said that he appealed to the instinctual priorities of managers as he 'sold' equal opportunity policy on the basis of 'good management practice' as 'most managers would agree with this' (142).

The use of pragmatic, or utilitarian, arguments for policy implementation was a central characteristic of the 'political economy' of equal opportunities in Britain in the 1980s and 1990s (see Mason and Jewson, 1992; Jewson and Mason, 1994). The alleged business, rather than moral, benefits of policy have been promoted, in large part because of a belief that managerial practices are more likely to be shaped by enlightened self-interest than a concern for social justice. Some officials and health service managers interviewed believed that appeals to morality alone are not enough to stimulate policy activity. Moral arguments for policy implementation according to one senior manager (109) appeal to the 'idealists' who are the 'innovators' in relation to equal opportunity policy. However, in their view, the 'innovators' cannot secure the commitment of others by employing solely moral arguments. Instead, they have to use a language that managers will listen to. For some participants in the policy process - such as the EOC - the strategy appears to have been expeditious when recognising the limitations of moral exhortation, although morality implicitly remained the primary concern.

## Note

1 The material used in this chapter draws from the Ph.D. research of one of the authors (see Iganski 1993b).

# 4 Is the 'Black Nurse' an 'Endangered Species'?

In the late 1980s some commentators believed that 'black' nurses in Britain were a 'dying species'. Young people of minority ethnic descent were allegedly being deterred from a nursing career by the discrimination, disadvantage and harassment experienced by their parents as health service workers. One pioneer of this view, Carole Baxter, argued that: 'the nursing profession is rapidly becoming a far less attractive career possibility for black and ethnic minority groups than it used to be. British-born black school-leavers are reluctant to expose themselves to the humiliation and degradation endured by their parents, relatives and the community as a whole' (1988: 25). Baxter concluded that the 'number of black and ethnic minority nurses within the National Health Service is therefore seriously on the decline'. The disappearance of the 'black nurse' by the year 2000 was even predicted unless remedial recruitment initiatives were taken (Pearson, 1987: 26). There was some evidential basis for this prediction. Anecdotal evidence (Lee-Cunin, 1989: 29) and limited statistical evidence (CRE, 1987) suggested that the number of black applicants to pre-registration training in nursing and midwifery was lower than would be expected when compared with the representation of minority ethnic groups in the population as a whole.

The predicted demise of the 'black nurse' was rooted in the belief about the deterrent effect of racial discrimination and disadvantage operating within the NHS. There is a substantial body of anecdotal evidence concerning racial discrimination at work in the health services which has been reviewed elsewhere (cf. Akinsanya, 1988; Kushnick, 1988; Beishon *et al.*, 1995) and discussed in chapter two of this book. Although much of the evidence is anecdotal, its cumulative weight does suggest that discrimination has been a common experience for many minority ethnic nurses and midwives as well as for would-be students.

In the context of past discrimination, we explore in this chapter whether black nurses have indeed been deterred from nursing as a career, by examining the national pattern of applications - and their outcome - from members of minority ethnic groups to pre-registration nursing and midwifery courses in England during the 1990s. We also explore whether discrimination potentially affects the selection process. Our analysis is confined to pre-registration training because at the time of writing there are no available national data on applications to post-registration training. We use two sets of data. The first, and more substantial, was provided by the English National Board for Nursing, Midwifery and Health Visiting (ENB) as part of a commissioned research project (Iganski *et al.*, 1998). The ENB, until recently, administered applications, through its Nurses and Midwives Central Clearing House (NMCCH). It recorded anonymised application form information in a database. Extract files from the database were produced for the research in Lotus format by the NMCCH, which we then converted to SPSS system files for analysis. The data cover applications made to all nurse education and training institutions in England in three consecutive years: 1st October 1993 to 29th September 1994 ('Fixed application period' 1 [Fap 1]); 1st October 1994 to 29 September 1995 (Fap 2); and 1st October 1995 to 29th September 1996 (Fap 3). Two types of data file were made available by the ENB. One contains information on individual *applicants* and the other relates to individual *applications*, of which any applicant may make up to four. The analysis we present here utilises the applicant files which, when combined, contain anonymised data on 54,194 individual applicants across the three fixed application periods. These files provide data on the ethnic group of applicants (self-classified by applicants using the 1991 Census categories, with the addition by the ENB of an 'Irish' category), age, gender, country and health service region of residence, educational qualifications, together with the outcome of each application. Whilst the validity of the Census categories used has been questioned in terms of the extent to which they reflect the diversity and fluidity of ethnic group identity (Sheldon and Parker, 1992), they do provide a minimal basis, and the best available, for workforce planning.

From September 1997 applications have been administered by the Nursing and Midwifery Admissions Service (NMAS), commissioned by the NHS Management Executive. Data for 1997-1998 and 1998-1999 published by NMAS, combined with additional data provided by the NHS Management Executive for 1999-2000, constitute our second data set. It is far more limited than the NMCCH data, but it does constitute the most up-to-date set of data at the time of writing.

Some caution needs to be exercised in interpreting the data provided in this chapter from the NMCCH database and from NMAS. The NMCCH, and its successor NMAS, have provided only partial recruitment channels for nurse education and training institutions, as large numbers of applicants apply directly to institutions. Such applicants have generally not been recorded on the databases, unless they are advised by the institution to which they have applied to apply through the central application process. The number of direct applicants as a proportion of all applicants varies considerably between institutions. In one of the eight nurse education and training centres used as case studies for the research – the Saltash Institute - the Academic Coordinator estimated that only around half of its applicants for pre-registration programmes were generated from its NMCCH Handbook entry, and pointed out to us that 'most of the institutions rely on direct applicants' (011). Similarly, the senior administrator responsible for recruitment at the Wembury Institute (034) estimated that approximately forty-five per cent of their applicants apply directly to the Institute. In contrast, the Deputy Dean at the Lipson Institute stated that they have historically relied on direct applicants to fill just five per cent of their contract numbers (023).

There are no nationally collected data on the ethnic group composition of applicants direct to institutions and data collection in our research institutions was variable. The eight institutions involved in the research either did not collect ethnic group data from direct applicants, or in the case of the Wembury Institute of Health, had only analysed data for a few isolated cohorts. Thus, whilst the applicant data we use in this chapter are limited, they constitute the most comprehensive national data set available. In addition, there were no suggestions raised in our research institutions that the ethnic group composition of direct applicants differs markedly from those who apply through the central application process, although that possibility must remain open.

## Ethnic Group of Applicants Compared with the Population in England

Both sets of data enable us to determine the degree of any under-representation of applicants from minority ethnic groups. We begin with a comparison against the population of all ages in England, rather than against the age cohort from which the applicants are drawn. This is because it is arguable that, as the health services are used across the complete life-span, the demographic distribution of health service users of all ages is the relevant point of comparison. The population in England also provides the relevant point of comparison for whilst there are no contractual obligations for nurses and midwives to work in the area in which they have trained, nurse education and training institutions are contracted by Regional Health Authorities for training places on the basis of local workforce planning estimates (Gerrish *et al..*, 1996: 117). Table 4.1 presents data on applicants to the NMCCH for each of the three 'fixed application periods' separately.[1]

Not all applicants to the NMCCH provided the required information but, amongst those who did, nearly nine per cent of applicants for the three fixed application periods combined classified themselves into one of the Black groups. There is a considerable gender difference, in that nearly eighteen per cent of male applicants classified themselves as Black compared with nearly eight per cent of female applicants. 'Black Africans' are strongly represented amongst both groups. More specifically it can be seen that in each of the Black groups, in each of the three fixed application periods, both females and males are over-represented amongst applicants when compared with the representation of the groups in the population in England. The 'Black African' group shows the largest degree of over-representation compared with the 'Black Caribbean' and 'Black Other' groups. Even if all of the applicants who omitted to specify their ethnic group were re-classified as 'White' on the highly unlikely assumption that they would have so classified themselves, the Black groups combined would still be over-represented. It should be noted, however, that the 'Black African' group would account for the bulk of the over-representation. In contrast, each of the Asian groups is under-represented amongst applicants, with one exception: Indian males are over-represented in each of the three fixed application periods. Female and male applicants who classified themselves as 'White' are also under-represented compared with the representation of the groups amongst the population of all ages in England.

**Table 4.1 Applicants to pre-registration training in nursing and midwifery by ethnic group and gender, 1993-1996** (column percentages)[a, b]

| | 1993/94 | | 1994/95 | | 1995/96 | | Pop[c] |
|---|---|---|---|---|---|---|---|
| | N | % | N | % | N | % | % |
| *Female* | | | | | | | |
| White | 12,788 | 89.3 | 12,651 | 87.8 | 10,579 | 83.1 | 94.0 |
| Black Caribbean | 229 | 1.6 | 281 | 2.0 | 217 | 1.7 | 1.1 |
| Black African | 695 | 4.9 | 819 | 5.7 | 713 | 5.5 | 0.4 |
| Black Other | 70 | 0.5 | 71 | 0.5 | 65 | 0.5 | 0.4 |
| Indian | 171 | 1.2 | 195 | 1.4 | 137 | 1.1 | 1.7 |
| Pakistani | 48 | 0.3 | 46 | 0.3 | 42 | 0.3 | 0.9 |
| Bangladeshi | 13 | 0.1 | 10 | 0.1 | 14 | 0.1 | 0.3 |
| Chinese | 33 | 0.2 | 38 | 0.3 | 25 | 0.2 | 0.3 |
| Irish | 4 | 0[d] | 32 | 0.2 | 757 | 5.9 | --[e] |
| Any Other Group | 277 | 1.9 | 270 | 1.9 | 218 | 1.7 | 1.0 |
| Total | 14,328 | 100.0 | 14,413 | 100.0 | 12,947 | 100.0 | 100.0 |
| *Not Specified* | *1,207* | *(7.8)* | *1,421* | *(9.0)* | *1,904* | *(12.8)* | |
| *Male* | | | | | | | |
| White | 1,753 | 74.9 | 1,778 | 72.1 | 1,575 | 71.6 | 93.6 |
| Black Caribbean | 32 | 1.4 | 31 | 1.3 | 28 | 1.3 | 1.0 |
| Black African | 341 | 14.6 | 405 | 16.4 | 308 | 14.0 | 0.5 |
| Black Other | 15 | 0.6 | 28 | 1.1 | 14 | 0.6 | 0.4 |
| Indian | 50 | 2.1 | 84 | 3.4 | 73 | 3.3 | 1.8 |
| Pakistani | 9 | 0.4 | 11 | 0.5 | 8 | 0.4 | 1.0 |
| Bangladeshi | 1 | 0 | 3 | 0.1 | 3 | 0.1 | 0.4 |
| Chinese | 6 | 0.3 | 3 | 0.1 | 4 | 0.2 | 0.3 |
| Irish | 2 | 0.1 | 3 | 0.1 | 83 | 3.8 | -- |
| Any Other Group | 131 | 5.6 | 119 | 4.8 | 105 | 4.8 | 1.0 |
| Total | 2,340 | 100.0 | 2,465 | 100.0 | 2,201 | 100.0 | 100.0 |
| *Not Specified* | *288* | *(11.0)* | *254* | *(9.3)* | *426* | *(16.2)* | |

a Column totals may not equal 100 due to rounding.

b Throughout the chapter we do not subject the data to tests of statistical significance as the data we use cover all applicants in the files, not samples of applicants. Observed differences are therefore actual differences, and not potentially due to sampling error.

c Population in England. Source: U.K. Office of Population Censuses and Surveys (1993), *1991 Census. Ethnic Group and Country of Birth. Great Britain*, vol. 2, HMSO, London, table 6.

d 0 indicates less than 0.05 per cent.

e -- indicates no applicants in this category, or no data in the case of population data.

Substantial proportions of applicants in each of the three fixed application periods were resident outside Great Britain at the time of their application (Table 4.2). Applicants living in England were asked to enter a code on their application form for the nearest Nurse Education and Training Institution (as indicated in the NMCCH applicant handbook). Applicants living outside England were asked to enter a code according to whether they lived in: Scotland, Wales, Northern Ireland, the Republic of Ireland, 'Other EEA' countries, or the 'Rest of the World'. For each of the ethnic groups there is some variation across the three fixed application periods in terms of the proportions resident outside Great Britain but there are some clear patterns. Amongst female applicants, those who classified themselves as 'Irish' have the highest proportions resident outside Great Britain at the time of their application. Amongst the other groups, the Black Caribbean, Black African, Indian, and Chinese groups have significant proportions resident outside Great Britain relative to the White group, whereas the proportions for the Pakistani and Bangladeshi groups are lower compared with Whites, although there are only a small number of applicants involved. For males, each of the Black and Asian groups – with the exception of the Bangladeshi group – consistently have far higher proportions than Whites across the three fixed application periods resident outside Great Britain. The proportions are also consistently higher than for female applicants from the groups concerned.

For the more recent data on applications administered by NMAS, applicants are asked to provide ethnic origin information only if their permanent residence is in the U.K. Therefore, they have not been included in our analysis so far. But from this point on we confine our analysis to GB resident applicants - or those resident in the U.K. in the case of the NMAS data. It seems reasonable to exclude overseas applicants from the discussion at this point because applicants resident in Great Britain would arguably be more likely to share cultural characteristics with communities resident in Britain than overseas applicants. This is a significant issue considering the links discussed in Chapter 3 between the recruitment of health service workers from minority ethnic communities and the provision of services sensitive to the needs of those communities.

Table 4.3 presents data on female applicants who were resident in Great Britain at the time of their application (GB applicants in the NMCCH data who classified themselves as 'Irish' are included from this point on in the 'White' group). It can be seen that each of the Asian groups remain under-

**Table 4.2 Percentage of applicants to pre-registration training in nursing and midwifery resident outside Great Britain, by ethnic group and gender, 1993-1996**

| | 1993/94 | | 1994/95 | | 1995/96 | |
|---|---|---|---|---|---|---|
| | %[a] | N[b] | % | N | % | N |
| *Female* | | | | | | |
| White | 6.5 | 12,370 | 5.9 | 12,131 | 1.1 | 10,109 |
| Black Caribbean | 30.0 | 210 | 30.8 | 214 | 24.1 | 174 |
| Black African | 24.9 | 611 | 25.6 | 632 | 22.1 | 521 |
| Black Other | 7.6 | 66 | 8.2 | 61 | 8.3 | 60 |
| Indian | 28.2 | 156 | 21.9 | 155 | 20.6 | 107 |
| Pakistani | -- | 46 | 2.3 | 43 | -- | 36 |
| Bangladeshi | -- | 13 | -- | 10 | -- | 14 |
| Chinese | 26.7 | 30 | 40.0 | 30 | 13.0 | 23 |
| Irish | 100.0 | 3 | 85.7 | 28 | 80.9 | 582 |
| Any Other | 30.1 | 246 | 16.5 | 231 | 18.1 | 193 |
| Total | | 13,751 | | 13,535 | | 11,819 |
| *Not Specified* | *7.6* | *459* | *11.9* | *1,108* | *7.1* | *911* |
| *Male* | | | | | | |
| White | 4.8 | 1,707 | 3.9 | 1,719 | 0.7 | 1,472 |
| Black Caribbean | 43.3 | 30 | 64.0 | 25 | 28.0 | 25 |
| Black African | 42.1 | 290 | 39.0 | 282 | 30.5 | 223 |
| Black Other | 50.0 | 14 | 29.2 | 24 | 55.6 | 9 |
| Indian | 56.1 | 41 | 56.3 | 64 | 54.9 | 51 |
| Pakistani | 50.0 | 4 | 20.0 | 10 | 16.7 | 6 |
| Bangladeshi | -- | 1 | -- | 3 | 33.3 | 3 |
| Chinese | -- | 5 | 100.0 | 2 | 75.0 | 4 |
| Irish | 100.0 | 2 | 66.7 | 3 | 47.0 | 66 |
| Any Other | 36.1 | 119 | 33.0 | 94 | 21.7 | 83 |
| Total | | 2,213 | | 2,226 | | 1,942 |
| *Not Specified* | *7.6* | *92* | *8.1* | *172* | *6.1* | *197* |

[a] Percentage of applicants in the group resident outside Great Britain.

[b] 'N' for each of the three fixed application periods represents the number of applicants who specified their country/region of residence.

represented compared with their representation in the population as a whole in England. The degree of under-representation is increased for the Indian and Chinese groups but is reduced for the Pakistani and Bangladeshi groups across both the NMCCH and NMAS data; although they remain under-represented. Amongst the 'Black' groups the representation of the Black Caribbean group is reduced, with a relatively small reduction for the 'Black Other' group, although each of the groups remains over-represented compared with their representation in the population. The over-representation of the Black African group is increased in the NMAS data. The White group remains under-represented but the degree of under-representation is reduced considerably.

For males (Table 4.4), the Indian group moves from over-representation (Table 4.1) to under-representation when applicants resident outside Great Britain are excluded, while the degree of under-representation is increased for the Pakistani and Chinese groups. There is some variable change for Bangladeshi applicants who remain under-represented. However, the numbers of applicants involved for each of these groups is very small. Amongst Black applicants, the Black Caribbean group moves to a position of under-representation, with a similar pattern for the Black Other group who are under-represented in two of the three fixed application periods in the NMCCH data, but they are slightly over-represented in the NMAS data. The representation of the Black African group is reduced considerably in the NMCCH data, although it remains significantly over-represented compared to its representation in the population as a whole, and it increases in the NMAS data. As is the case for female applicants, White male applicants remain under-represented but the degree of under-representation is reduced considerably.

It was argued above that the population in England, of all ages, provides the relevant comparison to determine under-, or over-, representation of the minority ethnic groups when issues of service delivery are being considered. However, labour supply considerations suggest an additional comparison against the age cohorts from which applicants are primarily drawn. Over three-quarters of applicants resident in Great Britain in each of the three fixed application periods were aged between 16 and 29 years. Data for this age group are presented in table 4.5 (we are again limited to the NMCCH data as the same age breakdown is not possible with the NMAS data). The data show that, when the comparison is restricted to this age group, the over-representation of some Black groups previously observed disappears, although those identified as Black African remain over-represented.

**Table 4.3 G.B. resident applicants* by ethnic group compared with the population in England, females, 1993-1996 and 1997-2000** (column percentages)

| | 1993/94 | | 1994/95 | | 1995/96 | | Pop |
|---|---|---|---|---|---|---|---|
| | N | % | N | % | N | % | % |
| White | 11,565 | 91.8 | 11,422 | 91.5 | 10,111 | 91.8 | 94.0 |
| Black Carib | 147 | 1.2 | 148 | 1.2 | 132 | 1.2 | 1.1 |
| Black African | 459 | 3.6 | 470 | 3.8 | 406 | 3.7 | 0.4 |
| Black Other | 61 | 0.5 | 56 | 0.5 | 55 | 0.5 | 0.4 |
| Indian | 112 | 0.9 | 121 | 1.0 | 85 | 0.8 | 1.7 |
| Pakistani | 46 | 0.4 | 42 | 0.3 | 36 | 0.3 | 0.9 |
| Bangladeshi | 13 | 0.1 | 10 | 0.1 | 14 | 0.1 | 0.3 |
| Chinese | 22 | 0.2 | 18 | 0.1 | 20 | 0.2 | 0.3 |
| Any Other | 172 | 1.4 | 193 | 1.6 | 158 | 1.4 | 1.0 |
| Total | 12,597 | 100.0 | 12,480 | 100.0 | 11,017 | 100.0 | |
| *Not specified* | *424* | | *976* | | *846* | | |

| | 1997/98 | | 1998/99 | | 1999/2000 | | Pop |
|---|---|---|---|---|---|---|---|
| | N | % | N | % | N | % | % |
| White | 12,190 | 91.1 | 18,295 | 88.3 | 18,057 | 86.0 | 94.0 |
| Black Carib | 172 | 1.3 | 294 | 1.4 | 343 | 1.6 | 1.1 |
| Black African | 544 | 4.1 | 1,255 | 6.1 | 1,600 | 7.6 | 0.4 |
| Black Other | 76 | 0.6 | 145 | 0.7 | 162 | 0.8 | 0.4 |
| Indian | 92 | 0.7 | 180 | 0.9 | 204 | 1.0 | 1.7 |
| Pakistani | 82 | 0.6 | 135 | 0.7 | 158 | 0.8 | 0.9 |
| Bangladeshi | 20 | 0.2 | 33 | 0.2 | 33 | 0.2 | 0.3 |
| Chinese | 18 | 0.1 | 33 | 0.2 | 38 | 0.2 | 0.3 |
| Any Other | 192 | 1.4 | 333 | 1.6 | 395 | 1.9 | 1.0 |
| Total | 13,386 | 100.0 | 20,703 | 100.0 | 20,990 | 100.0 | |
| *Not specified* | *2,501* | | *5,307* | | *6,750* | | |

* U.K. in the case of the NMAS data for 1997-2000.

**Table 4.4 G.B. resident applicants* by ethnic group compared with the population in England, males, 1993-1996 and 1997-2000**
(column percentages)

| | 1993/94 | | 1994/95 | | 1995/96 | | Pop |
|---|---|---|---|---|---|---|---|
| | N | % | N | % | N | % | % |
| White | 1,626 | 84.7 | 1,653 | 84.6 | 1,497 | 84.6 | 93.6 |
| Black Carib | 17 | 0.9 | 9 | 0.5 | 18 | 1.0 | 1.0 |
| Black African | 168 | 8.8 | 172 | 8.8 | 155 | 8.8 | 0.5 |
| Black Other | 7 | 0.4 | 17 | 0.9 | 4 | 0.2 | 0.4 |
| Indian | 18 | 0.9 | 28 | 1.4 | 23 | 1.3 | 1.8 |
| Pakistani | 2 | 0.1 | 8 | 0.4 | 5 | 0.3 | 1.0 |
| Bangladeshi | 1 | 0.1 | 3 | 0.2 | 2 | 0.1 | 0.4 |
| Chinese | 5 | 0.3 | -- | -- | 1 | 0.1 | 0.3 |
| Any Other | 76 | 4.0 | 63 | 3.2 | 65 | 3.7 | 1.0 |
| Total | 1,920 | 100.0 | 1,953 | 100.0 | 1,770 | 100.0 | |
| *Not specified* | *85* | | *158* | | *185* | | |

| | 1997/98 | | 1998/99 | | 1999/2000 | | Pop |
|---|---|---|---|---|---|---|---|
| | N | % | N | % | N | % | % |
| White | 1746 | 86.6 | 2719 | 82.4 | 2438 | 76.0 | 93.6 |
| Black Carib | 16 | 0.8 | 18 | 0.6 | 25 | 0.8 | 1.0 |
| Black African | 174 | 8.6 | 400 | 12.1 | 539 | 16.8 | 0.5 |
| Black Other | 9 | 0.5 | 22 | 0.7 | 19 | 0.6 | 0.4 |
| Indian | 13 | 0.6 | 24 | 0.7 | 34 | 1.1 | 1.8 |
| Pakistani | 5 | 0.3 | 6 | 0.2 | 17 | 0.5 | 1.0 |
| Bangladeshi | -- | -- | 1 | 0 | 1 | 0 | 0.4 |
| Chinese | 2 | 0.1 | 3 | 0.1 | 4 | 0.1 | 0.3 |
| Any Other | 52 | 2.6 | 107 | 3.2 | 129 | 4.0 | 1.0 |
| Total | 2,017 | 100.0 | 3,300 | 100.0 | 3,206 | 100.0 | |
| *Not specified* | *828* | | *3,095* | | *4,007* | | |

* U.K. in the case of the NMAS data for 1997-2000.

**Table 4.5 G.B. resident applicants by ethnic group and gender compared with the population in England, 16-29* year olds, 1993-1996** (column percentages)

| | 1993/94 | | 1994/95 | | 1995/96 | | Pop |
|---|---|---|---|---|---|---|---|
| | N | % | N | % | N | % | % |
| *Female* | | | | | | | |
| White | 9,485 | 92.2 | 9,458 | 92.4 | 8,070 | 92.8 | 92.9 |
| Black Carib | 102 | 1.0 | 95 | 0.9 | 73 | 0.8 | 1.3 |
| Black African | 364 | 3.5 | 339 | 3.3 | 278 | 3.2 | 0.6 |
| Black Other | 47 | 0.5 | 44 | 0.4 | 42 | 0.5 | 0.5 |
| Indian | 92 | 0.9 | 103 | 1.0 | 70 | 0.8 | 1.8 |
| Pakistani | 41 | 0.4 | 42 | 0.4 | 35 | 0.4 | 1.0 |
| Bangladeshi | 13 | 0.1 | 10 | 0.1 | 14 | 0.2 | 0.3 |
| Chinese | 18 | 0.2 | 12 | 0.1 | 13 | 0.2 | 0.4 |
| Any Other | 126 | 1.2 | 134 | 1.3 | 99 | 1.1 | 1.1 |
| Total | 10,288 | 100.0 | 10,237 | 100.0 | 8,694 | 100.0 | |
| *Not specified* | *330* | | *784* | | *646* | | |
| *Male* | | | | | | | |
| White | 1,204 | 84.6 | 1,273 | 86.2 | 1,095 | 86.9 | 92.5 |
| Black Carib | 14 | 1.0 | 8 | 0.5 | 13 | 1.0 | 1.3 |
| Black African | 119 | 8.4 | 113 | 7.7 | 75 | 6.0 | 0.7 |
| Black Other | 5 | 0.4 | 14 | 1.0 | 3 | 0.2 | 0.5 |
| Indian | 14 | 1.0 | 20 | 1.4 | 17 | 1.4 | 2.0 |
| Pakistani | 2 | 0.1 | 5 | 0.3 | 4 | 0.3 | 1.1 |
| Bangladeshi | 1 | 0.1 | 2 | 0.1 | 1 | 0.1 | 0.4 |
| Chinese | 5 | 0.4 | -- | -- | 1 | 0.1 | 0.4 |
| Any Other | 59 | 4.2 | 42 | 2.8 | 51 | 4.1 | 1.2 |
| Total | 1,423 | 100.0 | 1,477 | 100.0 | 1,260 | 100.0 | |
| *Not specified* | *58* | | *111* | | *132* | | |

* Age 30, for 1995/96, due to the age categories used for the database that year.

## Ethnic Group of Applicants by Training Specialism

Table 4.6 presents data on applicants - of all ages - resident in Great Britain according to the training specialism for which they have applied. At this point we have to confine our analysis again to the earlier NMCCH data for 1993-96 as the more recent data do not provide a breakdown by specialism.

Although they are often taught with a common foundation programme, each nursing specialism, as well as the midwifery specialism, constitutes a distinct area of work requiring specific skills. It is relevant, therefore, to treat the specialisms as different areas of work when evaluating patterns of under and over-representation. The data show that there is no uniform pattern of under-, or over-, representation for the minority ethnic groups across the main specialisms. Among females, White applicants are slightly under-represented in the main specialisms apart from mental health nursing, where there is a much larger degree of under-representation. Each of the Black groups is over-represented in all specialisms, with only one exception; Black Caribbeans are under-represented in Children's nursing (they are also only slightly over-represented in adult nursing). Children's nursing is the least popular overall with Black applicants but in contrast it is the most popular with applicants from each of the Asian groups. Among the Black groups, the over-representation of Black Africans is by far the most significant and this is especially the case for Mental Health nursing. The Asian groups are all under-represented in each of the specialisms.

Among males, White applicants are under-represented in each of the specialisms and the extent of under-representation is greater than that of White female applicants. The under-representation of White males is due to the strength of the representation of the minority ethnic groups combined and amongst them the strong over-representation of Black African males in each of the specialisms. This, in turn, is greater than the over-representation of female applicants from the same group, and especially so in mental health nursing where they constitute nearly one-sixth of all applicants. Male applicants who classified themselves as Black Other are also over-represented in three of the main specialisms: mental health, learning disability, and children's nursing, although the numbers of applicants involved are very small.

**Table 4.6 G.B. resident applicants by ethnic group, gender, and training specialism, compared with the population in England, 1993-1996** (FAPs 1,2 and 3 combined) (column percentages)

| | Mid-wifery | Adult | Mental Health | Learn. Disability | Child | Other | Pop |
|---|---|---|---|---|---|---|---|
| | % | % | % | % | % | % | % |
| *Female* | | | | | | | |
| White | 92.9 | 92.5 | 85.3 | 90.0 | 92.7 | 86.8 | 94.0 |
| Black Carib | 1.4 | 1.1 | 1.5 | 1.6 | 0.8 | 2.5 | 1.1 |
| Black African | 2.5 | 3.2 | 8.8 | 4.6 | 2.8 | 6.7 | 0.4 |
| Black Other | 0.8 | 0.4 | 0.8 | 0.8 | 0.4 | 0.4 | 0.4 |
| Indian | 0.8 | 0.9 | 0.7 | 0.5 | 1.1 | 0.6 | 1.7 |
| Pakistani | 0.4 | 0.3 | 0 | 0.5 | 0.6 | 0.1 | 0.9 |
| Bangladeshi | 0 | 0.1 | 0.1 | 0 | 0.2 | 0.1 | 0.3 |
| Chinese | 0 | 0.2 | 0.1 | 0.1 | 0.2 | 0.3 | 0.3 |
| Any Other | 1.2 | 1.3 | 2.5 | 2.0 | 1.1 | 2.4 | 1.0 |
| Total | 3,932 | 21,840 | 2,855 | 891 | 5,003 | 1,573 | 100.0 |
| Not specified | 287 | 1,268 | 201 | 61 | 311 | 118 | |
| *Male* | | | | | | | |
| White | 78.4 | 89.9 | 76.0 | 82.6 | 86.4 | 79.5 | 93.6 |
| Black Carib | 5.9 | 0.6 | 0.9 | -- | 1.6 | 1.1 | 1.0 |
| Black African | 9.8 | 4.6 | 15.9 | 11.0 | 6.8 | 11.8 | 0.5 |
| Black Other | -- | 0.4 | 0.7 | 0.4 | 0.7 | 0.8 | 0.4 |
| Indian | 2.0 | 1.0 | 1.4 | 0.4 | 1.3 | 3.0 | 1.8 |
| Pakistani | -- | 0.4 | 0.2 | -- | 0.3 | -- | 1.0 |
| Bangladeshi | -- | 0.1 | 0.1 | -- | -- | 0.4 | 0.4 |
| Chinese | -- | 0.1 | 0.2 | -- | -- | -- | 0.3 |
| Any other | 3.9 | 3.1 | 4.5 | 5.5 | 2.9 | 3.4 | 1.0 |
| Total | 51 | 3,086 | 1,698 | 236 | 309 | 263 | 100.0 |
| Not specified | 7 | 223 | 136 | 18 | 22 | 22 | |

## Application Outcomes

Table 4.7 presents NMCCH data for each of the three fixed application periods on applicants who had either commenced training, or having accepted an offer were waiting for a training place, when the NMCCH database files were downloaded for the research. The data show that White female and male applicants are consistently the most likely - when compared with the minority ethnic groups - to have commenced training, or be holding an offer of training. (The data for some minority ethnic groups, in some FAPs, do indicate higher rates of applicants in training or holding an offer of training compared with Whites. However, no reliable conclusions can be drawn because of the small numbers involved.) In addition, with a few exceptions, female applicants are generally more likely than male applicants to have commenced training or be holding an offer of training. Although there are evident differences among the minority ethnic groups, there are no other consistent patterns.

Table 4.8 presents data on the number and proportions of applicants in training, or holding an offer of training, by ethnic group for each of the three fixed application periods, compared with the population in England. When looked at from this further perspective, the data show that the minority ethnic groups that are over-represented among applicants, with the exception of Black Africans, decline to a position of near parity, or under-representation, compared with the respective group proportions of the population in England.

The more recent NMAS data on application outcomes show the same overall trend as the earlier NMCCH data, although with slightly more variation (Table 4.9). In general, White applicants are more likely to have a training place than applicants from the minority ethnic communities – with only a few exceptions: Black Caribbeans in 1997-1998, Pakistani males in 1998-1999 and Chinese males in 1999-2000, but the numbers in the last two groups are too small for a reliable comparison. Among White applicants, males are consistently more likely to have a training place than female applicants.

**Table 4.7 Applicants in training, or waiting to commence training, by ethnic group and gender, G.B. resident applicants, 1993-1996**

| | 1993/94 | | 1994/95 | | 1995/96 | |
|---|---|---|---|---|---|---|
| | N[a] | %[b] | N | % | N | % |
| *Female* | | | | | | |
| White | 6,507 | 56.3 | 6,264 | 54.8 | 6,404 | 63.3 |
| Black Carib | 68 | 46.3 | 58 | 39.2 | 80 | 60.6 |
| Black African | 100 | 21.8 | 95 | 20.2 | 133 | 32.8 |
| Black Other | 25 | 41.0 | 24 | 42.9 | 28 | 50.9 |
| Indian | 35 | 31.3 | 55 | 45.5 | 42 | 49.4 |
| Pakistani | 19 | 41.3 | 13 | 31.0 | 18 | 50.0 |
| Bangladeshi | 9 | 69.2 | 7 | 70.0 | 8 | 57.1 |
| Chinese | 8 | 36.4 | 7 | 38.9 | 12 | 60.0 |
| Any Other | 50 | 29.1 | 71 | 36.8 | 78 | 49.4 |
| Total | 6,821 | 54.2 | 6,594 | 52.8 | 6,803 | 61.8 |
| *Not specified* | *220* | *51.9* | *524* | *53.7* | *404* | *47.8* |
| | | | | | | |
| *Male* | | | | | | |
| White | 845 | 52.0 | 880 | 53.2 | 945 | 63.1 |
| Black Carib | 3 | 17.7 | 3 | 33.3 | 4 | 22.2 |
| Black African | 35 | 20.8 | 32 | 18.6 | 59 | 38.1 |
| Black Other | 2 | 28.6 | 4 | 23.5 | 1 | 25.0 |
| Indian | 4 | 22.2 | 6 | 21.4 | 5 | 21.7 |
| Pakistani | 2 | 100.0 | 3 | 37.5 | 3 | 60.0 |
| Bangladeshi | -- | -- | 3 | 100.0 | -- | -- |
| Chinese | 3 | 60.0 | -- | -- | -- | -- |
| Any Other | 20 | 26.3 | 19 | 30.2 | 36 | 55.4 |
| Total | 914 | 47.6 | 950 | 48.6 | 1053 | 59.5 |
| *Not specified* | *38* | *44.7* | *76* | *48.1* | *94* | 50.8 |

a N = the number of applicants in training, or waiting to commence training having accepted an offer.

b Percentage of the group in training, or waiting to commence training having accepted an offer.

**Table 4.8 G.B. resident applicants in training, or waiting to commence training, by ethnic group and gender, compared with the population in England, 1993-1996** (column percentages)

| | 1993/94 | | 1994/95 | | 1995/96 | | Pop |
|---|---|---|---|---|---|---|---|
| | N | % | N | % | N | % | % |
| *Female* | | | | | | | |
| White | 6,507 | 95.4 | 6,264 | 95.0 | 6,404 | 94.1 | 94.0 |
| Black Carib | 68 | 1.0 | 58 | 0.9 | 80 | 1.2 | 1.1 |
| Black African | 100 | 1.5 | 95 | 1.4 | 133 | 2.0 | 0.4 |
| Black Other | 25 | 0.4 | 24 | 0.4 | 28 | 0.4 | 0.4 |
| Indian | 35 | 0.5 | 55 | 0.8 | 42 | 0.6 | 1.7 |
| Pakistani | 19 | 0.3 | 13 | 0.2 | 18 | 0.3 | 0.9 |
| Bangladeshi | 9 | 0.1 | 7 | 0.1 | 8 | 0.1 | 0.3 |
| Chinese | 8 | 0.1 | 7 | 0.1 | 12 | 0.2 | 0.3 |
| Any Other | 50 | 0.7 | 71 | 1.1 | 78 | 1.2 | 1.0 |
| Total | 6,821 | 100.0 | 6,594 | 100.0 | 6,803 | 100.0 | 100.0 |
| *Not specified* | *220* | | *524* | | *404* | | |
| *Male* | | | | | | | |
| White | 845 | 92.5 | 880 | 92.6 | 945 | 89.7 | 93.6 |
| Black Carib | 3 | 0.3 | 3 | 0.3 | 4 | 0.4 | 1.0 |
| Black African | 35 | 3.8 | 32 | 3.4 | 59 | 5.6 | 0.5 |
| Black Other | 2 | 0.2 | 4 | 0.4 | 1 | 0.1 | 0.4 |
| Indian | 4 | 0.4 | 6 | 0.6 | 5 | 0.5 | 1.8 |
| Pakistani | 2 | 0.2 | 3 | 0.3 | 3 | 0.3 | 1.0 |
| Bangladeshi | -- | -- | 3 | 0.3 | -- | -- | 0.4 |
| Chinese | 3 | 0.3 | -- | -- | -- | -- | 0.3 |
| Any Other | 20 | 2.2 | 19 | 2.0 | 36 | 3.4 | 1.0 |
| Total | 914 | 100.0 | 950 | 100.0 | 1053 | 100.0 | 100.0 |
| *Not specified* | *38* | | *76* | | *94* | | |

**Table 4.9 Applicants in training, or waiting to commence training, by ethnic group and gender, U.K. resident applicants, 1997-2000**

| | 1997/98 | | 1998/99 | | 1999/2000 | |
|---|---|---|---|---|---|---|
| | N[a] | %[b] | N | % | N | % |
| *Female* | | | | | | |
| White | 8,468 | 69.5 | 10,524 | 57.5 | 9,974 | 55.4 |
| Black Carib | 121 | 70.4 | 145 | 49.3 | 176 | 51.3 |
| Black African | 284 | 52.2 | 372 | 29.6 | 486 | 30.4 |
| Black Other | 47 | 61.8 | 62 | 42.8 | 77 | 47.5 |
| Indian | 59 | 64.1 | 84 | 46.7 | 97 | 47.6 |
| Pakistani | 51 | 62.2 | 56 | 41.5 | 76 | 48.1 |
| Bangladeshi | 10 | 50.0 | 13 | 39.4 | 11 | 33.3 |
| Chinese | 11 | 61.1 | 18 | 54.6 | 14 | 36.8 |
| Any Other | 110 | 57.3 | 145 | 43.5 | 174 | 44.1 |
| Total | 9,161 | 68.4 | 11,419 | 55.2 | 11,085 | 52.8 |
| *Not specified* | *1,119* | *67.7* | *705* | *64.6* | *973* | 20.6 |
| *Male* | | | | | | |
| White | 1223 | 70.1 | 1562 | 57.5 | 1373 | 56.3 |
| Black Carib | 13 | 81.3 | 7 | 38.9 | 12 | 48.0 |
| Black African | 94 | 54.0 | 100 | 25.0 | 154 | 28.6 |
| Black Other | 3 | 33.3 | 11 | 50.0 | 4 | 21.1 |
| Indian | 8 | 61.5 | 11 | 45.8 | 19 | 55.9 |
| Pakistani | 2 | 40.0 | 4 | 66.7 | 7 | 41.2 |
| Bangladeshi | -- | -- | -- | -- | -- | -- |
| Chinese | 1 | 50.0 | 1 | 33.3 | 3 | 75.0 |
| Any Other | 31 | 59.6 | 37 | 34.6 | 58 | 45.0 |
| Total | 1,375 | 68.2 | 1,733 | 52.5 | 1630 | 50.8 |
| *Not specified* | *232* | *84.7* | *161* | *38.1* | *209* | 30.4 |

a N = the number of applicants in training, or waiting to commence training having accepted an offer.

b Percentage of the group in training, or waiting to commence training having accepted an offer.

## Explaining Differences in Application Outcomes by Ethnic Group

In the discussion of the outcome of applications above, we observed that White female and male applicants were consistently more likely to have commenced training, or be holding an offer of training, compared to the minority ethnic groups. Here we attempt to explain the pattern of differential outcomes. Again, our analysis is restricted to the NMCCH data, and it is further constrained from this point by limitations to the database records. It is not possible to determine precisely from either the application or the applicant data files every applicant, and every application, which received an offer of a training place. The application files are more seriously affected. Each applicant could apply to up to four institutions. When they accepted an offer from an institution, however, a code was automatically given to the institutions to which they had applied indicating that they had accepted an offer elsewhere (AE). It is not possible, therefore, to know whether or not applicants had been offered a training place in any institution apart from the one accepted.

Given limitations affecting the application files our analysis relies principally upon the applicant files. However, limitations also affect the applicant file. For instance, one category - or field - on the file, with a code (WE) which refers to applicants who withdrew their application, does not distinguish between applicants who withdrew before an offer might have been made and those who withdrew after an offer. The majority of applicants can be accounted for, but uncertainty affects a substantial number. This limitation is less substantial than the difficulty with the application files, hence our decision to limit our analysis to the applicant files. However, whilst we provide the most comprehensive data available, some caution needs to be exercised in interpreting them.

To permit a multivariate analysis with reliable numbers of applicants, the data for the three fixed application periods are combined. Data on whether applicants have commenced training, or are waiting to commence training having accepted an offer, are used as a surrogate for application outcome: the dependent variable. These are the most convenient data available on the NMCCH database in terms of which application outcome can be evaluated, given the limitations of the application file. The independent variables used for the analysis - in other words, those that might have an impact on application outcome - cover sex, age, ethnic group, educational qualifications, the training specialism to which applicants applied, and whether a visa was required. Our analysis is confined to applicants resident in Great Britain at the time of their application for reasons explained above. All of the independent variables, apart from the age variable, are nominal measures and consequently limit the multivariate analysis that might be applied. Given the limitations to the data, no attempt is made to measure the impact of each independent variable in combination with the others. Instead, the analysis is restricted to controlling for the impact of the independent variables in various combinations. The analytic strategy adopted, then, is not to seek to measure precisely how each variable contributes to outcomes but rather to identify the extent to which there are differences which remain unexplained when the effects of these variables are taken into account. This is in line with the aims of the original research commissioned by the ENB and has the additional merit of making the discussion accessible.

Our analysis addresses a fundamental question; when account is taken cumulatively of each of the independent variables, are there any unexplained differences in application outcome between Whites and the minority ethnic groups which might suggest that discriminatory processes (whether intentional or unintentional) are at work in the selection of applicants for training in nursing and midwifery?

### *Differences in Educational Qualifications*

One key potential explanatory variable could be differences in the level of educational qualifications held by members of different groups. Outcome differentials might be explained if members of some groups were relatively less likely to hold the minimum qualifications necessary for admission to nursing and midwifery training. Alternatively if, on average, the qualification levels of members of some groups were lower than others, they might be at a disadvantage if the levels of qualification required for entry by particular institutions exceeded the minimum set by the ENB. The Commission for Racial Equality, in a mail survey carried out in the late 1980s (see Chapter 2), identified a lower success rate for black applicants relative to others for entry to nurse training, although with far more limited data than that presented here. The CRE observed that: 'Given what is known from the Swann Report about the academic achievement levels of

Afro-Caribbean youths, it is likely that they will be disproportionately rejected or discouraged from applying for admission to nursing schools by academic requirements which may not in fact be necessary for successful completion of the training course' (CRE, 1987: para. 14).

The first of these explanations does not apply in the case of our data, since all those recorded on the NMCCH database satisfied the minimum requirements for entry into nursing and midwifery training. In other words, all applicants on the database were eligible for entry. There are, however, clear differences between White applicants and some of the minority ethnic groups in terms of the distribution of educational qualifications (Table 4.10). For female applicants, for the three fixed application periods combined, 75.5 per cent of the White group hold 'traditional' academic qualifications of GCSEs, A Levels, Diploma, or a Degree. This compares to 34.7 per cent of Black Caribbeans, 29.7 per cent of Black Africans, and 47.1 per cent of those who classified themselves as Black Other. There is a much smaller differential between Whites and the Asian groups, and the Bangladeshi group has marginally more (75.9 per cent) applicants with traditional academic qualifications than White females, but the comparison is unreliable as Bangladeshi applicants are very few in number. A similar pattern can be observed when White males as a group are compared with males from each of the minority ethnic groups. If nurse education and training institutions use a hierarchy of educational qualifications above the minimum set by the ENB as selection criteria, then differences in the distribution of qualifications between ethnic groups might be expected to lead to group differences in the outcome of applications.

To determine whether the observed differentials affect the application outcomes between the groups, it is necessary to control for group differences in educational qualifications. To do this we compare each of the groups in each qualification band, in terms of whether they were in training, or waiting to commence training having accepted an offer, at the time the database records were downloaded for the research (Table 4.11).

With a few exceptions, smaller proportions of the minority ethnic groups are successful in their applications than White applicants in the same qualification bands. In other words, males and females from each of the minority ethnic groups are less successful than Whites, even when controlling for educational qualifications.

**Table 4.10 Educational qualifications by ethnic group and gender, G.B. resident applicants** (Faps 1,2 and 3 combined) (row percentages)

| | Dipl. /degree | A levels | 5+ GCSE | 5 GCSE | BTEC | GNVQ | NVQ Level 3 | Access | DC Test | Prev reg | Other |
|---|---|---|---|---|---|---|---|---|---|---|---|
| *Females* | | | | | | | | | | | |
| White | 3.9 | 22.5 | 34.3 | 14.8 | 9.2 | 0.5 | 0.7 | 3.0 | 3.6 | 0.1 | 7.5 |
| Black Carib | 6.1 | 10.8 | 9.6 | 8.2 | 17.1 | 0.5 | 0.7 | 23.8 | 2.1 | -- | 19.2 |
| Black African | 2.8 | 7.9 | 11.1 | 7.9 | 6.4 | 0.1 | 0.4 | 7.8 | 1.4 | -- | 54.2 |
| Black Other | 4.1 | 14.0 | 16.8 | 12.2 | 16.3 | -- | 1.2 | 11.1 | 4.1 | -- | 20.4 |
| Indian | 3.5 | 19.8 | 22.3 | 16.4 | 16.1 | -- | 0.9 | 6.0 | 0.6 | -- | 14.5 |
| Pakistani | 3.2 | 21.8 | 33.1 | 14.5 | 16.1 | 0.8 | -- | 4.8 | 0.8 | -- | 4.8 |
| Bangladeshi | -- | 10.8 | 48.7 | 16.2 | 18.9 | -- | -- | 5.4 | -- | -- | -- |
| Chinese | 6.7 | 20.0 | 15.0 | 3.0 | 13.3 | -- | -- | 8.3 | -- | -- | 31.7 |
| Other | 4.6 | 20.1 | 17.8 | 9.0 | 5.0 | 0.2 | 0.2 | 3.4 | 4.8 | 0.2 | 34.8 |
| All Groups | 3.9 | 21.7 | 32.7 | 14.4 | 9.2 | 0.4 | 0.7 | 3.5 | 3.8 | 0.1 | 9.9 |
| *Males* | | | | | | | | | | | |
| White | 9.6 | 25.8 | 19.1 | 11.2 | 8.5 | 0.2 | 0.4 | 3.1 | 9.6 | 0 | 12.3 |
| Black Carib | 6.8 | 4.6 | 11.4 | 6.8 | 6.8 | -- | 2.3 | 11.4 | 11.4 | -- | 38.6 |
| Black African | 3.4 | 12.5 | 12.9 | 7.7 | 2.4 | -- | -- | 2.2 | 1.0 | -- | 37.8 |
| Black Other | 3.6 | 35.7 | 17.9 | 3.6 | 3.6 | -- | -- | 7.1 | 3.6 | -- | 25.0 |
| Indian | 4.4 | 24.6 | 10.2 | 14.5 | 8.7 | 1.5 | -- | 1.5 | 5.8 | -- | 29.0 |
| Pakistani | 13.3 | 20.0 | -- | 6.7 | 20.0 | -- | -- | 6.7 | -- | -- | 33.3 |
| Bangladeshi | -- | 50.0 | -- | -- | -- | -- | -- | -- | -- | -- | 50.0 |
| Chinese | -- | 50.0 | -- | -- | -- | -- | -- | -- | 16.7 | -- | 33.3 |
| Other | 7.8 | 21.1 | 10.8 | 10.3 | 4.4 | -- | -- | 1.0 | 10.8 | -- | 33.8 |
| All Groups | 8.8 | 24.4 | 18.0 | 10.8 | 7.8 | 0.2 | 0.5 | 3.0 | 8.8 | 0 | 17.6 |

**Table 4.11 Proportions of G.B. resident applicants, by educational qualifications, ethnic group and gender, who are in training, or waiting to commence training** (Faps 1, 2 and 3 combined)

| | Dipl. /degree % | A levels % | 5+ GCSE % | 5 GCSE % | BTEC % | GNVQ % | NVQ Level 3 % | Access % | DC Test % | Prev reg % | Other % |
|---|---|---|---|---|---|---|---|---|---|---|---|
| *Females* | | | | | | | | | | | |
| White | 58.4 | 60.7 | 59.9 | 53.1 | 63.0 | 74.2 | 59.6 | 64.5 | 43.7 | 40.9* | 47.2 |
| Black Carib | 19.2* | 52.2 | 43.9 | 51.4 | 52.1 | 100.0* | 66.7* | 63.6 | 22.2* | -- | 32.9 |
| Black African | 56.8 | 23.6 | 23.0 | 22.9 | 33.7 | 100.0* | 40.0* | 51.9 | 36.8* | -- | 18.1 |
| Black Other | 85.7* | 37.5* | 55.2* | 23.8* | 64.3* | -- | 50.0* | 52.6* | 57.1* | -- | 22.9 |
| Indian | 45.5* | 41.3 | 47.9 | 36.5 | 51.0 | -- | 66.7* | 63.2* | 50.0* | -- | 15.2 |
| Pakistani | 25.0* | 48.2* | 41.5 | 27.8* | 40.0* | 100.0* | -- | 33.3* | 100.0* | -- | 33.3* |
| Bangladeshi | -- | 75.0* | 61.1* | 83.3* | 71.4* | -- | -- | 0* | -- | -- | -- |
| Chinese | 50.0* | 75.0* | 88.9* | 33.3* | 50.0* | -- | -- | 40.0* | -- | -- | 5.3* |
| Other | 41.7* | 40.0 | 45.2 | 36.2 | 53.9* | 0 | 0* | 72.2* | 28.0* | 0* | 29.7 |
| All Groups | 57.3 | 59.6 | 59.1 | 51.9 | 61.6 | 74.4 | 59.0 | 62.9 | 43.3 | 39.1 | 39.2 |
| *Males* | | | | | | | | | | | |
| White | 61.1 | 59.6 | 57.2 | 51.6 | 64.6 | 80.0* | 57.1* | 66.7 | 39.2 | 0* | 50.2 |
| Black Carib | 33.3* | 0* | 40.0* | 0* | 33.3* | -- | 100.0* | 20.0* | 20.0* | -- | 17.7* |
| Black African | 35.3* | 29.0 | 18.8 | 15.8 | 25.0* | -- | -- | 45.5* | 0* | -- | 26.6 |
| Black Other | 100.0* | 30.0* | 0* | 0* | 100.0* | -- | -- | 0* | 100.0* | -- | 14.3* |
| Indian | 33.3* | 47.1* | 0* | 10.0* | 16.7* | 100.0* | -- | 100.0* | 0* | -- | 10.0* |
| Pakistani | 100.0* | 100.0 | -- | 0* | 0* | -- | -- | 100.0* | -- | -- | 40.0* |
| Bangladeshi | -- | 66.7* | -- | -- | -- | -- | -- | -- | -- | -- | 33.3* |
| Chinese | -- | 66.7* | -- | -- | -- | -- | -- | -- | 0* | -- | 50.0* |
| Other | 50.0* | 48.8 | 31.8* | 23.8* | 66.7* | -- | -- | 100.0* | 27.3* | -- | 29.0 |
| All Groups | 59.7 | 57.5 | 53.5 | 47.3 | 62.4 | 81.8* | 58.6* | 63.9 | 37.8 | 0* | 40.2 |

The analysis is limited by the small numbers of applicants from some of the minority ethnic groups across the different qualification bands, making comparison unreliable for the bands concerned. Hence the discussion from this point - and the corresponding analysis - is limited to an evaluation of qualification band by ethnic group where there are more than thirty applicants in a band (cells in the tables with less than thirty applicants are marked *). Despite the limitations of such an analysis, the data clearly show differential outcomes for the minority ethnic groups concerned, which cannot be explained away by differences in educational qualifications.

For female applicants, it can be seen that the Black Caribbean, Black African and Indian groups each have fewer successful applicants compared to Whites in each qualification band where numbers of applicants enable a reliable comparison. Overall, the Black African group shows the largest differential relative to Whites. Male applicants from the Black African group are also less successful than Whites at each qualification level where a reliable comparison can be made.

*Training Specialism*

The training specialism to which applicants applied provides a further variable that we controlled in analysing ethnic group differentials in application outcomes. If a specialism exhibits a greater demand for training, in terms of the number of applications relative to training places, this would result in a higher proportion of unsuccessful applicants compared to other specialisms. If, in addition, an ethnic group has a higher proportion of applicants to that specialism compared with other ethnic groups, then differential application outcomes may be explained away by the pattern of applications.

If we take female applicants from the Black African, Black Caribbean and Indian groups combined, applicants to midwifery have the lowest success rate (27.4 per cent), followed by applicants to the Child branch (45.1 per cent), with the Adult, Mental Health, and Learning Disability branches falling in a very narrow range between 60.7 per cent and 61.9 per cent. The effect of these differential success rates between the specialisms appears to be minimal, marginally affecting the Black Caribbean group, which has the highest proportion of applicants to midwifery, and the Indian group which has the highest proportion of applicants to the Child branch.

However, an evaluation of the application success rates by ethnic group and qualification band indicates that the pattern of differential application outcomes between Whites and the selected minority ethnic groups remains, and cannot be explained away by different success rates between the branches. Proportions of applicants in training, or waiting to commence training, by ethnic group, training specialism, and educational qualifications, are provided in Table 4.12. (The analysis is further confined to female applicants from this point, due to the unreliability of using the small number of male applicants for this more detailed analysis.) The analysis reveals the limitations of the data as the small number of applicants in the majority of cells prevents reliable comparison. However, in each of the cells where it is possible to make a comparison, the minority ethnic groups are less successful in every instance. The analysis is limited but it indicates a persistent differential between the minority ethnic groups concerned and the White group in terms of application outcomes which cannot be explained away by a combination of group differences in educational qualifications and patterns of applications across the training specialisms.

*Visa Requirements*

Although all of the applicants used for the analysis in this chapter were resident in Great Britain at the time of their application, an examination of the database reveals that some of them are recorded as requiring a visa if they were successful in their application to training in nursing or midwifery. It is, in principle, possible that in some institutions such applicants might be rejected, either because it might be assumed that they would not be able to obtain a visa, or that an application for a visa might add an unwanted complication to the selection process. It is therefore necessary to control for those applicants requiring a visa. However, removal of applicants requiring a visa from the base numbers has little impact on group differentials in application outcomes as differences remain for the selected groups in each qualification band. In most cases minority

**Table 4.12 Proportions of G.B. resident applicants, by ethnic group, training specialism and educational qualifications, who are in training or waiting to commence training, 1993-1996** (females only, Faps 1, 2 and 3 combined)

| | Midwifery | Adult | Mental Health | Learning Disability | Child |
|---|---|---|---|---|---|
| *White* | | | | | |
| Diploma/Degree | 47.3 | 62.6 | 58.4 | 56.5 | 47.6 |
| BTEC | 27.9 | 69.5 | 68.4 | 74.3 | 49.3 |
| Access | 43.4 | 69.2 | 72.4 | 58.8 | 50.0 |
| A Levels | 34.4 | 66.6 | 68.6 | 63.4 | 51.5 |
| 5+ GCSE | 24.7 | 67.2 | 65.3 | 63.0 | 50.3 |
| 5 GCSE | 19.6 | 59.4 | 59.0 | 68.9 | 36.4 |
| Other | 22.3 | 49.5 | 61.6 | 54.4 | 35.4 |
| *Black Caribbean* | | | | | |
| Diploma/Degree | 9.1* | 20.0* | 100.0* | -- | -- |
| BTEC | 30.0* | 53.9 | 50.0* | 50.0* | 70.0* |
| Access | 40.0* | 61.5 | 70.0* | 80.0* | 75.0* |
| A Levels | 50.0* | 51.7* | 50.0* | -- | 66.7* |
| 5+ GCSE | 33.3* | 50.0* | 20.0* | -- | 16.7* |
| 5 GCSE | 66.7* | 62.5* | 33.3* | 100.0* | 33.3* |
| Other | 33.3* | 28.0 | 66.7* | 33.3* | 0* |
| *Black African* | | | | | |
| Diploma/Degree | 0* | 73.3* | 55.6* | 100.0* | 25.0* |
| BTEC | 0* | 35.0 | 58.3* | 0.0* | 22.2* |
| Access | 33.3* | 56.9 | 38.1* | 50.0* | 50.0* |
| A Levels | 14.3* | 21.7 | 27.6* | 28.6* | 10.0* |
| 5+ GCSE | 21.4* | 24.3 | 24.1* | 33.3* | 15.8* |
| 5 GCSE | 0* | 17.0 | 28.0* | 25.0* | 26.7* |
| Other | 1.7 | 14.0 | 32.8 | 47.6* | 11.7 |
| *Indian* | | | | | |
| Diploma/Degree | 33.3* | 25.0* | 100.0* | -- | -- |
| BTEC | 25.0* | 55.0 | 100.0* | -- | 33.3* |
| Access | 100.0* | 64.7* | -- | -- | 0* |
| A Levels | 14.3* | 21.1 | 50.0* | 0* | 40.0* |
| 5+ GCSE | 44.4* | 52.6 | 40.0* | 100.0* | 37.5* |
| 5 GCSE | 20.0* | 45.5* | 25.0* | 100.0* | 31.6* |
| Other | 100.0* | 12.1 | 20.0* | 0* | 25.0* |

* indicates a base number for the cell of less than 30 applicants.

ethnic applicants are less successful than Whites, and in a number of qualification bands the differences remain considerable, especially for the Black African group.

*Age*

The age of applicants provides a last available variable that might potentially explain the observed group differences in application outcomes. If particular age groups of applicants are more successful in their applications relative to others, then the different age profiles of the groups might explain group differences in application outcomes. In line with the analytic strategy adopted for this chapter, the aim is not to measure the contribution made by age differences to application outcomes, but to control for age in order to determine whether differential outcomes persist. A simplified way of doing this is to take one age band (16-25 year olds), one qualification band (5+ GCSEs, which has the largest number of applicants amongst the qualification bands), and compare the relative success rates of the selected ethnic groups. The relevant data are presented in Figure 4.1 and Table 4.13. It can be seen that even when controlling for age, considerable differences are evident between Whites and the selected groups in the same qualification band. The differences cannot, therefore, be explained away by age and qualification level combined. In line with the preceding analysis, the greatest differential is evident for the Black African group.

## Conclusions to Be Drawn From the Data

The data in this chapter provide the most comprehensive evaluation to date of patterns of applications to training in nursing and midwifery by ethnic group, and show complex patterns of representation, among applicants, of Whites and the minority ethnic groups, and of women and men within the groups. Whilst some caution needs to be exercised about the data, a number of significant patterns emerge. The arguments about the importance of proportional representation which rely upon service delivery considerations suggest that the key comparitor is numbers of applicants in each ethnic group relative to the population as a whole. Looked at from this point of view, among females – constituting the great majority of

**Figure 4.1 Percentage of 16-25 year old female G.B. resident applicants in qualification band '5 GCSEs or more', by selected ethnic group - in training, or waiting to commence training**

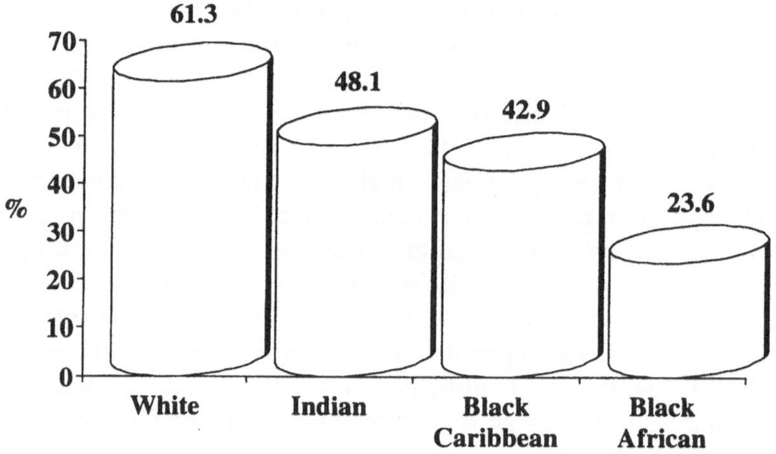


**Table 4.13 Numbers of 16-25 year old female G.B. resident applicants in qualification band '5 GCSEs or more', by selected ethnic group - in training, or waiting to commence training**

| | White | | Indian | |
|---|---|---|---|---|
| | N[a] | T[b] | N | T |
| 16-25 | 9,803 | 6,010 | 52 | 25 |
| All ages | 11,086 | 6,659 | 65 | 30 |
| | Black Caribbean | | Black African | |
| 16-25 | 28 | 12 | 106 | 25 |
| All ages | 41 | 18 | 146 | 34 |

a N = number of applicants.
b T = number of applicants in training, or waiting to commence training.

applicants – each of the Black groups has been consistently over-represented, with a very strong degree of over-representation for the Black African group. Amongst male applicants there has been no single pattern for the Black groups but Black African males have been even more strongly over-represented than female applicants from the group. The pattern of over-representation declines when the comparitor is the population aged between sixteen and twenty-nine. The pattern for females and males in each of the Asian groups is very clear. They are consistently under-represented amongst applicants for training in nursing and midwifery - across each of the specialisms.

The data on patterns of applications show, however, that whilst the discrimination experienced by earlier generations of the black nurses in the NHS may have a deterrent effect on potential black applicants for training in nursing and midwifery - and, as shown in Chapter 2, some of our respondents believed this to be the case - it does not appear to be a sufficient deterrent to lead to an under-representation of the groups amongst applicants compared to their representation in the population as a whole in England. In short, the data on applications show that predictions about the demise of the 'black nurse' which rely upon interpretations of the intentions of young people within the black groups may have been premature. Unless, that is, applications from the groups concerned were significantly higher in the 1980s compared with the levels shown by the data above. There are, however, no equivalent data for the earlier period to determine whether this might have been the case.

We should note that the predictions about the demise of the 'black nurse' often used the term 'black' inconsistently. Sometimes it appears to be used as a generic surrogate for 'minority ethnic'. On other occasions, formulations like 'black and ethnic minorities' are used. We use the term here in the limited sense in which it is embodied in Census and ENB classifications. If the Asian groups are subsumed under one homogeneous 'Black' category, as has been the practice in some of the earlier literature, the representation of the 'Black' group amongst applicants relative to the population declines considerably. This does not, however, support the deterrent-effect hypothesis as there is little evidence that 'Asian' minorities have ever been anything than under-represented.

The data on applications to training in nursing and midwifery indicate that processes appear to be operating within some Asian communities that result in a poor interest in nursing or midwifery as a career - expressed in terms of applications. Our data represent the aggregate choices of young people from the communities concerned. Whether the pattern of choices is a consequence of cultural factors, collective career aspirations, or other reasons, the under-representation of the Asian communities amongst applicants to training in nursing and midwifery provides a matter of concern in view of the connections made between ethnic diversity in the nursing and midwifery workforce and the provision of health services sensitive to the needs of minority ethnic communities.

When we turn to the outcome of applications there are further concerns with regard to each of the Black and Asian minority ethnic groups. All those minority ethnic groups whose numbers are large enough to permit conclusions to be drawn are less likely - when compared with White applicants - to have commenced training, or be holding an offer of training. When compared with the population as a whole, moreover, those groups previously over-represented among applicants, with the exception of Black Africans, decline to a position of near parity or under-representation amongst those in training, or holding an offer of training. Moreover, for the minority ethnic groups whose numbers permit an appropriate analysis, there are evident differences - which in some cases are substantial - in terms of having commenced training, or holding an offer of a training place, compared with White applicants which cannot be explained by the data. This suggests that factors may be at work in the selection process which are discriminating against some applicants on the basis of their ethnic group. In the next chapter we focus on selection practices by drawing on our qualitative research.

## Note

1 Unfortunately, it is not possible to provide a reliable time-series analysis across the three years of NMCCH data. The database file for a fixed application period continued to be updated after the end of the period as applicants with offers outstanding either commence training or withdraw, after the end of the period in which they applied. The interval between the end of the FAP and the date on which the file was downloaded for the research was different for each period. Whilst they are close, each FAP is at a different stage in terms of data processing. A comparison between the ethnic groups

within a FAP is perfectly valid, however, as there would be no reason to suggest that any observed differences between the groups in terms of application outcome would be due to the stage of data processing. For the NMAS data it is possible to compare application outcomes year-by-year as the data represent the full application year.

# 5 Selecting Applicants for Training in Nursing and Midwifery

Chapter 4 shows that there are differences in the success rates of applicants for pre-registration nursing and midwifery training that cannot be explained solely by reference to the characteristics of the applicants themselves. There has been little research to date on the extent to which the selection systems utilised by nurse education and training institutions accord with the principles of fairness and equity normally associated with effective equal opportunities policies.[1] Accordingly, this chapter focuses on the processes used by nurse education and training institutions for the selection of applicants for training in nursing and midwifery.

The equal opportunities literature is replete with recommendations about measures designed to provide equity and fairness in selection. Although most recommendations have been developed in relation to selection for employment, it can be argued that the same basic principles apply to selection for educational training and, hence, to training in nursing and midwifery. In essence, conventional recommendations emphasise a number of elements. First, it is characteristically argued that fair and equitable systems require selection criteria which are consistent, open and justifiable, in the sense that they are defined by reference to the tasks which successful applicants will be required to perform. Second, systems are required that ensure that the criteria are, and are seen to be, consistently applied to all candidates. Third, where selection comprises a number of stages, arrangements are needed to ensure that fairness, in the application of selection criteria, operates at each stage. This characteristically implies that, fourthly, a limited number of, ideally specially trained, personnel are involved in the selection process. Fifth, records of decisions, justified in terms of selection criteria, are necessary in order to permit the periodic review and auditing of decision-making.

## Selection Processes: The King's Fund Recommendations

A major source of equal opportunity recommendations focusing specifically on the health service can be found in the reports of the King's Fund Equal Opportunities Task Force. These focus primarily upon selection for employment but they have clear implications for nurse education and training.

### *Person Specifications*

The King's Fund Equal Opportunities Task Force recommended that person specifications, designed to provide clear and agreed criteria for selection, should be used for shortlisting and interviewing for employment in the health services. Criteria concerning, for example, experience and educational qualifications should match the elements of the job description. They should avoid additional requirements which cannot be shown to be necessary and that could form the basis of direct or indirect discrimination under the 1975 Sex Discrimination Act and the 1976 Race Relations Act (KFEOTF, 1987: 9-12). The objective, in other words, is that all job applicants be considered solely on the basis of their ability to do the job. It is not difficult to see how this process could be adapted for the selection of candidates for nursing and midwifery training. The aim would be to ensure that applicants are selected solely on the basis of merit – that is, with regard to their ability successfully to complete the course. For this to be possible, training courses would require to be evaluated to determine the educational and other pre-requisites necessary for successful completion. Selection criteria could then be formalised which match these pre-requisites. Whether or not they are formally labelled as person specifications these criteria would be used for initial sifting, shortlisting and interviewing of applicants. In its recommendations for selection procedures for hospital doctors, the King's Fund Equal Opportunities Task Force (1990: 9) further recommended that members of selection panels should be able to see and comment on criteria before they are expected to apply them. It also recommended that Directors of Personnel should check job descriptions and person specifications. In the same way, it could be argued that, in nurse education and training institutions, a senior member of staff should be allocated responsibility for overseeing the selection of students and monitoring the use of selection criteria.

*Shortlisting and Interviewing*

The King's Fund Equal Opportunities Task Force further recommended that, in order to secure the consistent application of selection criteria, shortlisting and interviewing should be carried out by the same panel of more than one person with representation, whenever possible, from the personnel department. Moreover it recommended that only those trained in the appropriate skills should be involved (KFOETF, 1987: 9-12). The aim of this recommendation is to reduce the intrusion of subjectivity, and to promote consistency, in selection decisions. There are clear parallels in the case of the selection of applicants to training in nursing and midwifery. It is arguable that the initial sifting of applications, shortlisting and interviewing should similarly be carried out by the same panel of more than one person; again with representation from the senior manager whose responsibility it is to oversee the implementation of equal opportunities policy.

*Training and Guidance*

Staff involved in selection processes obviously occupy a central role in relation to the provision of equal opportunities at work. Accordingly, the King's Fund Equal Opportunities Task Force recommended that *everybody* involved in the recruitment and selection of staff should receive recruitment and selection training within six months of appointment (KFEOTF, 1987: 9). Because of the significance of their role it is arguable that all staff involved in recruitment processes should receive *mandatory* training.

The Task Force (KFEOTF, 1987: 9-10) recommended that such training should cover:

- an exploration of the effects of assumptions and prejudices on selection decisions,
- the nature of discrimination,
- misunderstandings that might occur when interviewing candidates from different cultural backgrounds,

- the employee's liability under relevant legislation and the employer's own equal opportunities policy.

With regard specifically to interview panels, the Task Force (KFEOTF 1990: 10) also recommended that written guidance be provided to all panel members covering:

- the legislation and codes of practice,
- the legal liability of panels,
- ensuring selection according to agreed criteria,
- avoiding the use of informal visits, unsolicited references and patronage for selection decisions,
- unacceptable questions,
- procedures to follow if there are grounds for believing that discrimination may have taken place.

It has also been recommended that senior staff should receive training to develop understanding of their role in the employer's equal opportunities policy. This is particularly important, it is argued, if a serious commitment to equal opportunities within an organisation is to be developed (GLARE, 1987: 35). Equal opportunities training may also be appropriate for staff other than senior managers and those involved directly in recruitment processes. Other staff frequently occupy a significant gatekeeping role, as was demonstrated by the Commission for Racial Equality's formal investigation of St Chad's Hospital (CRE, 1984b) which concluded that discrimination against black applicants for domestic work had occurred. In this case, recruitment for domestic work relied upon casual inquiries that were dealt with in the first instance by telephonists or receptionists. It was alleged that these staff had been instructed by a manager to inform black inquirers that there were no vacancies. The case suggests that staff who deal with such inquiries need to be informed about their own liability under the relevant legislation and under their employer's equal opportunities policy.

## Selection Policy and Practice in Nurse Education and Training Institutions

To investigate selection policy and practice, we made a purposive selection of nurse education and training institutions in England, using a number of selection criteria to maximise the value of the sample in regard to our research objectives. From initial data produced in the statistical analysis of applicants and entrants to pre-registration training presented in Chapter 4, we ranked all 67 nurse education and training institutions in England relative to the others on the basis of the numbers of minority ethnic applicants they attracted. We confined selection of the institutions to those above the median. This criterion was applied to ensure that the selected institutions actually had some experience in administering applicants from minority ethnic groups. We then additionally ranked institutions above the median on the basis of the success rates, in terms of being offered a training place, of the minority ethnic groups combined. Financial resources available for our research project limited our final sample to eight nurse education and training institutions, determined by the estimated cost of the fieldwork. We selected four institutions from among those with the highest success rates of minority ethnic applicants, and four from those with the lowest. This second selection criterion was applied on the principle that higher success rates might indicate relatively more comprehensive or effective equal opportunity practice which could serve as an exemplar for other institutions. Similarly, lower success rates might indicate policy gaps that could also inform policy development. Such a criterion was clearly speculative but the aim was to elicit a variety of experience to inform policy development. We used a third and final criterion for the selection of the institutions, ranked, as explained on the basis of the other two criteria. Institutions were purposively selected on the basis that they were located in areas of above average minority ethnic residence and were distributed in a variety of geographical locations around England. The rationale for this criterion was that arguments for the achievement of an ethnically diverse workforce - and, by implication, cohorts of students in training - based upon the need for health care services sensitive to minority ethnic communities, would be particularly relevant for such institutions. It might be expected, therefore, that the selected centres would be more likely to use recruitment initiatives targeted at minority ethnic groups than centres in localities with lower than the national average representation of minority ethnic communities.

The purposive selection of a small sample of institutions using the selection criteria just described rules out any possibility of making generalisations from the research findings to all nurse education and training institutions in England. However, as each centre is located in an area with higher than the national average representation of minority ethnic communities, we might expect that the centres selected would be among the most active in developing equal opportunity measures. The selected centres might therefore reasonably be expected to offer lessons (whether positive or negative) for other nurse education and training institutions.

*Selection of Respondents Within Case Study Centres*

We sent a letter to the Head of each of the selected institutions explaining the aims of the proposed research and requesting a meeting to explore the possibility of using the centre as a case study site. One of the eight institutions initially selected declined this exploratory meeting and a replacement was selected from the reserve list. Eight centres agreed to participate in the research following the first meeting.

Heads of institutions were approached, in the first instance, on the basis that they had the authority to approve the participation of their centres. Their strategic positions also enabled them to sketch out an initial organisational plan, identifying for us the key individuals with prime responsibility for shaping, implementing and effecting recruitment and selection practices. The individuals identified in this way provided the initial respondents. Each respondent was subsequently asked to identify whom they regarded as the key individuals involved in the recruitment and selection processes, as a means of validating the initial list of potential respondents, and as a means of ensuring that all key respondents were included in the research. Managers with overall responsibility for selection were further asked to identify lecturers who were frequently involved in interviewing applicants. From the lists provided, we purposively selected potential respondents representative of the different training specialisms for nursing and midwifery. Interviews with these respondents sought to validate the descriptions of selection processes previously provided to us, and to evaluate whether there were any aspects of the selection processes that might prove vulnerable to the intrusion of unfair or discriminatory practices. In total, 81 respondents were interviewed for the research.

*Lines of Inquiry for the Research into Selection Policy and Practice*

In order to investigate selection policy and practice in the eight case study nurse education and training institutions, the Heads of each, together with the senior managers with overall responsibility for selection, were first asked to 'talk us through' the processes by which applicants are selected for training. The aim was to evaluate whether the processes used by the institutions had incorporated the policy guidance offered by bodies like the King's Fund Equal Opportunities Task Force and whether there were areas of selection practice where there was the potential for unfair practice or discrimination to occur.

The King's Fund recommendations discussed above suggested a number of lines of enquiry for the research. In relation to selection criteria, the researchers were keen to ask:

- *Are clear, open and consistent criteria drawn up for the selection of applicants?*
- *Are selection criteria formulated with regard to educational or other pre-requisites necessary for training programmes?*
- *Who draws them up?*
- *Can members of selection panels negotiate about the criteria prior to shortlisting and interview?*
- *Are these criteria explicitly used when sifting, shortlisting and interviewing applicants, and do they remain fixed during selection panel deliberations?*
- *Is there a senior member of staff whose responsibility it is to check the content and use of selection criteria used in shortlisting and interviewing?*

Turning to shortlisting and interviewing, the research sought to answer the following questions:

- *Who is responsible for shortlisting and interviewing?*
- *Are the same persons involved at each stage?*
- *Is there any requirement that persons involved in shortlisting and interviewing should have undergone equal opportunities or recruitment and selection training?*
- *Are all applications processed at the same time, or over a period of time?*
- *If applications are processed over a period of time, are the same selection criteria utilised on each occasion?*

With regard to training, the key lines of enquiry were:

- *Is training provided for staff shortlisting and interviewing applicants?*
- *Is training mandatory for all staff involved in shortlisting and interviewing?*
- *Is training provided for senior managers in nurse education and training institutions?*
- *Is training provided for other staff, such as telephonists, receptionists and administrators, who might deal with informal inquiries?*
- *What does the training cover?*
- *How often is training updated?*
- *Are those involved in the shortlisting and interviewing of applicants satisfied with the level and frequency of training received?*
- *Are those involved in selection procedures given written guidelines on selection practices?*

From some of the data provided by the ENB – and used in Chapter 4 – we observed that higher proportions of applicants from the minority ethnic groups compared with Whites were unsuccessful. More specifically, it appears that these higher rates of rejection were concentrated at the shortlisting stage of selection for pre-registration training. The application file records the stage in the selection process at which those applicants who are unsuccessful are rejected by institutions; either before or after interview. Table 5.1 provides the relevant data by ethnic group for G.B. resident females and males combined for fixed application period two, 1994-1995. Each applicant could apply on one application form to up to four nurse education and training institutions. The number of applications to institutions thus far exceeded the number of applicants. The data show clearly that there is little difference between the groups in the proportions of applications rejected following interview, and for some of the minority ethnic groups the proportions rejected are marginally lower than Whites. However, the data for those rejected before interview, at the shortlisting stage, are very significant. For each of the minority ethnic groups compared to Whites, higher proportions of applications were rejected without an interview and in some cases the differences are substantial. Such differences cannot be explained away by the observed limitations to the dependent variable used to represent application outcome – as discussed in Chapter 4.

**Table 5.1 Applications from G.B. residents by ethnic group rejected at shortlisting, or following interview (males and females combined), ENB data 1993-1996**

| | Stage of rejection | | | | |
|---|---|---|---|---|---|
| | Before interview | | After interview | | All applications |
| | N | % | N | % | N |
| White | 13,299 | 27.8 | 2,145 | 4.5 | 47,860 |
| Black Caribbean | 305 | 43.0 | 27 | 3.8 | 710 |
| Black African | 2,102 | 57.8 | 132 | 3.6 | 3,637 |
| Black Other | 136 | 40.5 | 18 | 5.4 | 336 |
| Indian | 279 | 39.9 | 32 | 4.6 | 699 |
| Pakistani | 64 | 32.3 | 9 | 4.6 | 198 |
| Bangladeshi | 15 | 28.9 | 2 | 3.9 | 52 |
| Chinese | 25 | 35.2 | 3 | 4.2 | 71 |
| Other | 604 | 47.0 | 49 | 3.8 | 1,284 |
| Total | 16,829 | 30.7 | 2,417 | 4.4 | 54,847 |
| *Not specified* | *1,237* | 29.6 | 157 | 3.8 | 4,185 |

In view of this, a key focus for the discussion in this Chapter will be the shortlisting and interview stages, the character of the personnel involved and the application of selection criteria at these respective stages. For the most part, applicants for *post*-registration courses were recommended by their employing trusts. In most cases, little action was required of institutions so far as selection was concerned. Nevertheless some applicants, particularly for longer courses, were subject to an interview process. This raised the same issues as those pertaining to pre-registration courses.

## A Case Study of a Formalised Selection Process

In only one of the case study institutions did it appear that concern about selection outcomes had given rise to a review of practice that had begun systematically to address the kinds of recommendations discussed above. Accordingly this evaluation of selection processes begins by focusing on the experience of an institution which had radically changed its procedures some years before the fieldwork for the research was carried out.[2] The change had been prompted by concerns about the efficiency of the selection processes in the context of high attrition rates of students but also motivated by suspicions that discrimination might have been occurring. With regard to discrimination, the Head of the Institute had observed a similar pattern of differential outcomes for applicants to the Institute as had been shown in Chapter 4 for applicants through the NMCCH. Applicants from the black and Asian minority ethnic groups were less successful overall in their applications compared to whites:

> when we looked at the sort of ethnic make up of the students who had applied, something was happening in the organisation that was precluding those students from getting either shortlisted, or if they were shortlisted, successfully interviewed in a manner that didn't meet up with the actual numbers of students who actually got as far as applying to us. So, we never got down to the root cause of what was happening, and why anything was happening because we didn't rush it too far. There was quite clearly a difference between the numbers of students applying and the numbers who made it to the starting grid ... whatever we were doing seemed to be working against them, now whether it was overt or covert I don't know.

The Administration Manager with overall responsibility for recruitment at the Institute made a similar observation:

> I think we were very concerned about our shortlisting because at that time we received many more applications for fewer places so there had to be some shortlisting and we weren't happy about the way it was being conducted by too many people. We did have some criteria but we weren't happy that it was consistent and then again at the interview stage it's open again to the usual sort of prejudice and we did some work to show we felt that male people for instance were not getting into the system, for whatever reason, so we were concerned about that ... (there was some) evidence that certain groups were discriminated against, males for instance particularly, just because of who happened to be shortlisting and who happened to be interviewing on the day it seemed. So we weren't satisfied with that.

The principal change had entailed the introduction of a telephone interviewing system that was well established by the time that the fieldwork was carried out. Senior staff in the institution were convinced that the changes had produced a transformation in the composition of the student cohort recruited, although no monitoring data were available which could conclusively have demonstrated this. Nevertheless, the Head of the Institute was convinced that change had occurred, observing that:

> it was clear from looking at the cohort that there seemed to be a richer mix of ethnic minority people, that's the subjective gut response from just looking at the group.

Shortlisting is carried out by administrative staff. However, at this stage only one criterion is used. Thus every applicant who meets the minimum educational qualifications specified in the Institute's NMCCH Handbook entry is offered an interview. The Administration Manager explained that:

> that was the area that caused concern before because there were a variety of people who were shortlisting, so there's no shortlisting going on so everybody has the opportunity to be interviewed ... everybody who applies is offered an interview so if they make an

> application they're offered an interview so we don't make any discriminating judgements there.

The interview process is highly standardised:

> It's all telephone, we don't do any face to face ... In fact we had one person who turned up, he got confused, so all we did, we put him in the meetings room and the lecturer rang him and no we don't do face to face ... I think it's about 18 people who do those interviews. All they do is they give the recruitment administrator a certain number of sessions when they will be available and she arranges interviews with students. All those interviewers receive is a form with the student's name, the telephone number, and the time and dates they're to ring them, so they don't know anything about the person ... And then each student is asked exactly the same question. The interview is a structured interview with 54 questions and it's tape recorded and so as I say I feel that does address a lot of the concerns about equal opportunities and we don't make any judgements about the academic qualifications they come in with. Obviously they meet the minimum and then the second part of the process is this interview.

On the basis of their responses in the interview, each candidate is given a score and candidates rated above a particular threshold are offered a training place:

> You either hit the target, in other words you give the correct response or you don't so you get a yes or a no, and then they're scored in themes, caring is one and we tot them all up so there's a score, below which at a certain level we wouldn't accept anybody. And then we also, we do a profile of the person. We plot that on what they call an ideograph so you can see the sort of balance of qualities that people have got, and we write a brief report, to say for instance this person scored very highly on caring and whatever, but is quite low on whatever and may need some support in prioritising or whatever and we think that is very useful information for personal teachers to have about a student, so rather than say find out in 18 months that the person perhaps doesn't show much attention to detail, they're aware

> that it's a possible feature of the personality from day one, so I think the information gleaned is invaluable.

The score required for success in the interview can be varied according to the recruitment needs of the institution:

> They strongly recommend that you don't accept people below a certain level and then there are bands so you get the sort of A plus people, the As and the Bs and you can see where the people you've accepted fall. Now, who you accept then is determined by the numbers you want for your contract, if you're only looking for small numbers then perhaps you could accept all the A pluses and with those you would expect that you've got the very best, so to some extent it's influenced by the numbers that you want. There's that balance between getting the numbers for your contracts and getting the right people, but below a certain level we wouldn't accept them.

All of the interviews are recorded, serving a number of purposes. First, interviewers can re-play the interview to check the accuracy of their rating. Second, and most importantly for equal opportunities purposes, the interviews are available for external scrutiny of the application of the questions and of the reliability of ratings given. Third, the recording provides evidence of the interview which may be utilised in the event of a complaint:

> the interviewers are trained to listen for a certain response that tells them whether the individual has that quality, but you can imagine that some candidates who you are interviewing are very easy, they're very clear and some are not quite so easy so the interviewer may want to play the tape again to decide and if it's a particularly difficult one and they're say just on the borderline they may want to ask a colleague to listen and score it. The other reason for tape recording is that we had the training from the Gallup organisation and to monitor standards we have to send them so many tapes and they check that the coding is up to scratch. And the third reason is that, that's a sort of quality control thing and the third reason is that if somebody who was refused made a complaint then again somebody else could listen to it, there's clear

> evidence and one of the questions that doesn't, they don't get a mark for this but at the end of the interview one of the questions asked them sort of how they felt about the interview so it gives them a chance to say oh fine or I didn't like it or whatever and in the situation where somebody felt they hadn't been treated fairly for instance, again you've got firm evidence of how they felt on the day and what they said.

The selection criteria, and the questions asked by the interviewers, are designed to remove, so far as possible, the potential for bias on the part of interviewers, and the subjective interpretation of responses:

> What we had before, we had areas where we would want tutors, lecturers to question students about, say for instance study skills, but we weren't more prescriptive than that. So it would be open to individuals to formulate the questions and then make a judgement on what they heard. And the other sort of prejudices that we were concerned about are the sort of things like the halo effect where people make a judgement on someone's appearance when they see them immediately and often, so the research says, they don't ... they make the decision and look for confirmation of it after that in what they hear and it sometimes, even the prejudices are subconscious about certain groups that can influence the decision and it's that sort of stuff that we wanted to get rid of if we could ... In those sort of face to face interviews people always think they're a good judge of other people and the evidence is that they're not. If you ask a person if they're good at something whatever, well of course they'll say yes, and many people don't have the interviewing skills to probe that further, and make a judgement so I don't think it was a very good way of doing things.

## Selection Practices in Other Case Study Institutions

By contrast with this relatively formalised and thought-through process, our research found considerable variation of practice elsewhere.[3]

### *Shortlisting*

The research revealed evidence of considerable variation in shortlisting practices and criteria across the institutions. Three different approaches to shortlisting could be found across the remaining institutions. Shortlisting was carried out either by an administrator, by a senior member of the academic staff – such as a branch leader – or by an administrator and member of the academic staff working together. In two of these approaches, one person alone is making judgements about the suitability of applicants. This may be a matter of some concern since, where selection criteria are very generalised, there is considerable scope for capricious or even overtly discriminatory decision-making when decisions are entrusted to individuals working alone. The Administration Manager at the Saltash Institute of Health explained their procedure:

> once they've got the minimum (educational qualifications) then that's fine. Obviously if they haven't we don't go past that first page on the application form. But normally if we get application forms from the NMCCH, most of it is fine because they check it first anyway. It doesn't always work like that because sometimes we find that they've sent things through and people haven't had the right qualifications, but that's how it's supposed to work but we still check it here. It's the direct application forms we have to be a bit more careful because obviously these are people that are just applying, some of them don't even know what the requirements are because they didn't get the pack or the book ... So it's the educational qualifications, that's the first thing, and the other thing we look for is their ... the supportive evidence, because we like people to at least have, even though they've never worked before, to just have some sort of insight on paper as to what, even if it's just I nursed my grandmother when she was ill, anything that looked ... like they have some sort of insight ... So those

are the two main things...if they leave that supportive evidence blank we're not interested (022).

When asked whether there were specific kinds of 'supportive evidence' that were sought, the same manager observed that:

> No, there isn't anything specific, as long as we read through and it sounds like they want to do nursing and like I said they don't have to have had any experience but just I've always wanted to be a nurse, even that, you know, that alone, that sort of thing. Just somebody that ... they have to sound like they want to do nursing on paper, I don't know how to explain it actually. I mean (the person carrying out the shortlisting) has been here for about seven years so she knows what to look for (022).

Shortlisting was carried out by a variety of individuals at the Peverell Institute, even within the same branch, although compared to Saltash, the criteria appear to be rather less indeterminate. The Adult Branch Leader explained that:

> Shortlisting's done by the subject leaders, but that is probably going to change in the near future because we do have thousands of applicants and certainly with the adult branch it's quite difficult. I have two people identified to help me shortlist but I do feel that the quality of shortlisting can only be contained if I have a small number shortlisting. The shortlisting criteria are the same for all branches and in the future, probably from about the autumn we hope that the registry staff will actually shortlist, mainly because our shortlisting criteria is about to become just academic qualifications and age ... At the moment it's academic qualifications, age, health record (026).

The Senior Administrator at the Mannamead Institute of Health did much of the shortlisting herself but also shortlisted together with academic staff. In some instances, academic staff carried out the shortlisting alone:

> I get all the forms, so they all come here ... We actually have criteria and it applies across the board, but if we look at the branches

> individually, the way we will do it is the lecturer and I will sit down together, go through the forms and we read every form and I know in some schools they put the details in the computer and do a random selection, but we read every form that comes in and we will shortlist probably down to about 40 or 50 from that under them criteria and we will interview over two or three days with service managers ... With the mental health it's a similar set up but the senior lecturer also likes to involve his teaching staff ... for learning disability, again the senior lecturer and I would look at the forms, now normally what happens is that what he says is that unless somebody has a dreadful application and a dreadful reference he will see them. So in lots of cases we don't sit down and look at them together, I look at the form and if there's something that's glaringly dreadful, I take it to him and we'll look at it together and decide, but really you know, the stance he takes, if somebody's bothered to apply then unless they've done something dreadful like they've come out of prison, like the person last week or whatever, then we would see them ... But then with the adult because you've got far bigger numbers and you've got two intakes in a year and the difference between courses is everybody applies has at least got the minimum qualifications ... so again I sit and I do an initial screening, I look through every form and again if there's something that's glaringly a problem they go on one side, if you've got a straightforward application that meets the criteria, support and information, references, there's no way that you wouldn't interview somebody, then it is a case of arranging an interview. The others that are not quite straightforward then I sit down with the senior lecturer and have a look at them (003).

When academic staff carry out the shortlisting themselves, the senior administrator vets any decisions to reject applicants:

> what I say is if you're not going to interview somebody we have to know, it has to be specific why ... But if anybody is not being interviewed it must be recorded on the form ... (one) member of staff always loves to do this, will send me a list of ... an A4 piece of paper with names on and reasons, but won't write them on so I do it, I go through them all and I write it on the back and I keep the notes, I said

> why don't you write it on the form you know and I don't know what it is, whether they think somebody's going to come back and take them to the tribunal or something, but what's the difference in writing it on a piece of paper and keeping it so the decision is written (003).

*Interviewing*

By contrast with the variations in shortlisting practice, between and within the case study institutions, there appeared to be a much greater degree of consistency with respect to interviewing practices. To a large extent, the kinds of policy measures embodied in the discussion of the King's Fund recommendations above were practised across the case study institutions. An example of a highly standardised telephone interview procedure in one institution has already been discussed. In the other institutions all interviews were carried out in person by a panel of more than one interviewer; normally with representation from service staff. Pre-determined selection criteria were used and a record made of the candidate's performance with regard to the questions asked. The only divergence from the equal opportunity policy recommendations across the institutions was that the same staff were generally not involved in shortlisting and interviewing. However, despite the formalisation of interview arrangements, there remained a considerable degree of discretion in most cases concerning the way that questions were asked and the interpretations made of the answers. By contrast with the script of standardised interview questions and scoring system described above, none of the other case study institutions had standardised procedures to the same extent. We were, therefore, interested in the range of discretion available to interviewers and the potential this left that such discretion might open the way for unlawful discrimination, whether conscious or unintentional.

Some respondents argued for the use of set questions by interviewers, specifically to reduce the scope for subjective biases. One interviewer from the Devonport Institute suggested that:

> I think what you've got to ask yourself is what actually are we assessing here and to what level are we assessing it and if there isn't a standardisation to that approach and if people are asking different questions of different people in different ways then there is no way of

> actually measuring that assessment apart from an individual intuitive point of view. And so it becomes a nonsense really (018).

Similarly, another interviewer from the Devonport Institute believed that:

> These questions were there to be asked in the same way, same manner to all applicants and that, in a way, I suppose is one way of being equal, you know, so I don't suppose they needed to justify that. In fact it was justified that everybody is getting equal you know, opportunity. It's only when you start to probe, there might be some difficulties for some people ... I think it's consistency, that one might come one day and get interviewed by someone else and may get asked different questions ... (016).

Other interviewers argued that they would feel too restricted by such a highly standardised system:

> what would be the point of making say a principal lecturer go through this process of reading from a pre-printed list of questions, putting them to this candidate and getting, it really makes you a machine and I wouldn't like to be put in that situation, what questions to ask and what answers to expect (061).

One institution, the Peverell Institute of Health, had specifically rejected a system of set questions, for reasons that the Adult Branch Leader explained:

> We started off with lists of questions years ago and we decided that was very restrictive, you have got to be able to go with the flow and we found that some interviewers were just sticking with the questions and maybe they would turn somebody down and when you talk to these people afterwards the whole thing had been just so rigid that whatever the answer had been wasn't then followed on, they were sticking to this list of questions so now we just have a broad concept of ways in which you could assess the elements we're looking for (026).

However, within the same Institution, a principal lecturer had developed a list of questions on her own initiative in an attempt to improve consistency in the application of selection criteria:

> when I came here I found the service side of great difficulty in interpreting that question regarding equity between different interview candidates, so what I've done is I've put together, which I'll run off now, two little questionnaires, one for education and one for service ... there were different questions and also different interpretation on the questions and sometimes people would miss questions out and I felt that some individuals weren't being asked consistently the same questions between each of the candidates, so to try and get some consistency in that. That's why I drew up these little questions, they're purely for me and it just supplements that criteria, that's all and I keep them (054).

However, the Adult Branch Leader at the Mannamead Institute of Health rationalised the use of discretion by interviewers by suggesting a value for subjective impressions:

> there are certain things that you can't ... certain things that you can't specifically look for but then you, by the things, the answers that they give you, the content about the things that they say, you get an overall feel for their attitude, their enthusiasm, their motivation and whether they actually really want to do this and what problems they think they might have along the way. I suppose really a sort of gut feeling for the individual (061).

However, a Lecturer in the Peverell Institute revealed the way that discretion on the part of interviewers might disadvantage applicants from some minority ethnic groups:

> A typical example is; 'what does your husband think?' I don't think we are going to ask a somebody from indigenous population white British woman 'what does your husband think of you coming to do nursing', but because we are aware of the problems particularly from the Asian student and their views of their husband and we do ask such

question. I think it is inappropriate ... That's just one typical example (049).

Interviewers in all of the case study institutions were required to make a record of the candidate's performance at interview, either with a written record, or numerical score, against different selection criteria. However, interpreting the answers provided by candidates leaves considerable potential for discretion on the part of the interviewer, especially when the selection criteria are not sufficiently specific:

> I think it's a matter of someone's own interpretation of the answers they receive, whether I feel happy that someone meets the criteria or if it doesn't, that not meeting is so severe as to cause me concern that whether we should consider this person at all ... I know some of them are ticked as essential and so on, but even with those, you need to use your … I think subjective imagination in deciding someone doesn't fully demonstrate that, whether that means automatically they should not be considered or the other way round, when someone does demonstrate that they have that particular quality but some of the other things that come with it that cause concern, that there is a problem here (061).

Similarly, another respondent asked:

> When is a 4 a 5 and when is a 3 a 4? I mean for example one of the criteria is 'experience in caring', well they may have experience in caring say but three years ago but you've got to mark them for that experience, so do you give them a one or a two depending on what they say and if someone's say got experience but been in the job say three months and want to do their nurse training, again where do you value that, 2 or 3? And also what they say and do, some may work in a group home but just stay in a group home all day, some work in the same group home but go out all the time, social education, so is that a three or a four so I find it very nebulous to be honest, I mean as long as I'm satisfied that they've got the experience and they want to do this level of nursing then I score them usually a four because they're

> committed to it, but it's very difficult to have hard and fast criteria for saying well this equals a one and this equals a two (054).

*Training and Guidance*

The importance of training was emphasised by the comments of a selector in the institution that had taken most steps to improve selection practice. Speaking of an earlier period our informant remarked:

> And some of us haven't had anything at all, and some people said it was on the job learning and some people said they were able to sit in and see somebody else do it so there was that. We weren't managed, there wasn't a person who directed us either, so given that we hadn't .... We didn't have the knowledge that we should have had, we then didn't have somebody who guided us in a particularly helpful way. We were very much left to our own devices and so what happened with that was not having had any background in the equal ops legislation, we then were able to apply our own set of criteria to everything that we did and so all sorts of subjective things were there (029).

Each of the case study institutions required staff to have undergone some form of equal opportunity or recruitment and selection training before they could be involved in interviewing applicants. There was, however, little evidence of systematic up-dating of the training after the initial training had been completed, and for some staff the time lapse was considerable:

> I have a long time ago, it was before the university, we joined the university, it was whilst I was teaching at the school of nursing, I went on a two day recruitment and selection course (070).

The on-going guidance given to staff around selection practices was also patchy across the eight case study institutions. For one lecturer, this left staff involved in interviews uncertain about how to apply the selection criteria:

the confusion that we have, some difficulty we have is really in relation to not having any guidance, I have no problem with it because I do use my subjective imagination but some people have a problem that if an essential criteria has not been met, whether that means even if it's one not met you could not possibly take this person in, irrelevant of how good the rest of the interview is, so people look at these ticks and worry sometimes you know, some one essential criteria has not been met, partially met or whatever, does that mean we cannot take this person or not and often when I led panels I used to get that question put to me, you know, can we take him, he doesn't fully meet this criteria and we don't seem to have written guidelines or policy in relation to them which may be a good thing, I'm not sure (061).

*Audit and Review*

Even in the institution which had taken the greatest steps to review its procedures, and where decision making was subject to careful review, there was evidence that systematic audit of the effectiveness of the selection and equal opportunities system was still some way off. It was noted above that no monitoring data were available to check whether the changes introduced had been effective.[4] More generally, respondents themselves could see scope for more systematic and regular reviews of various aspects of the system.

I think one of the most important things is when this three day equal opportunity is given to interviewers, I think there should be a limit, a period of time after which an evaluation is done to see what we are doing, how well we are not doing here, when the whole idea was to be able to recruit and retain people from ethnic minorities and be fair and avoid conflict, with ethnic minorities employees and I cannot recall when any evaluation has been made because if you ask me now have we made improvement from five years or six years ago of what the situation was regarding recruitment of ethnic minority I can't tell you. Maybe the authority will be able to tell you but I doubt it (049).

The importance of auditing selection decisions was stressed by a lecturer involved in interviewing at the institution that had introduced the telephone interviewing system:

> Nobody ever checked up to see how we'd done, who we'd rejected, why we'd rejected them, comparing shortlister to shortlister or comparing us at the beginning of the day to the end of the day even, there wasn't any sort of tight monitoring of what was going on and I think that given what I've already told you, I think that some people obviously have got some real problems with prejudice ... let's say everybody's been trained to the same standard, you've then got one individual who's making sure that the standards are adhered to all the time, and I mean in teaching this keeps coming up again and again, to me it reminds me of the marking that we do. If you haven't got somebody bringing it all together, and moderating it, the marking's all over the place, you've got to have somebody who keeps bringing us back to where we started, because we are all prejudiced and we have all got problems with certain things and I think if we don't. If we're not careful, that they can just come out, whether we're doing it deliberately or not.

In some of the other case study institutions, all applications rejected after interview were supposed to be monitored. However, in one instance, the manager responsible for the monitoring believed that interviewers should be responsible for their decisions:

> I don't want to get interviewers and tell them what they should be turning down and are they doing it professionally, because otherwise the quality of the whole thing becomes difficult to ... I am sometimes concerned, yes, sometimes say yes to people, sometimes I say no to people, but that is their decision and we have to respect it (011).

An admissions tutor similarly observed difficulties in challenging selection decisions:

> It's extremely difficult isn't it, because at the end of the day what actually goes down on paper may be different to the reason, the true

> reason why a candidate's been rejected and it's this whole issue I think between these gut feelings and these thinking feelings. And it may well be that somebody has a very strong feeling that this person is not going to be right and rejects them and applies the person specification to fit that rejection, but without being there within the interview itself it's very very hard to see that and to evaluate that ... I think it's also extremely difficult because as far as our heads of school are concerned, interviewing for courses is a responsibility for all teaching staff, so in theory by saying that, it's very hard for me to challenge my colleagues, my peers, my professional decisions that they've made (022).

## Conclusion

Overall, this chapter has revealed a mixed picture so far as the development of good equal opportunities practice within the case study institutions is concerned. While none of the institutions required educational qualifications in excess of the minimum for entry, there was evidence of the intrusion of other, often very general and unspecified criteria, at both shortlisting and interview stages. The shortlisting stage appears to be one that is particularly vulnerable to variations of practice between selectors and to the intrusion of a range of potentially discriminatory criteria. This had been explicitly recognised by the institution that had taken the greatest steps to review procedures.

Institutions had generally appeared to have responded to the basic recommendations reviewed above regarding interviewing. Nevertheless, respondents reported, sometimes with approval, that subjective decisions on a range of criteria remained possible. Only one institution had sought systematically to remove this scope by formulating a tightly structured interviewing instrument. Even here, it might be argued that the telephone interviewing process was vulnerable to the criticism that not all applicants have guaranteed access to a telephone in a location and environment which would allow them to perform at their best. However the system was, at least designed to remove many of the opportunities for subjectivity, discretion and caprice to which other systems were recognised by respondents themselves to be vulnerable.

So far as other aspects of good practice are concerned the picture is extremely mixed. Few institutions appeared systematically to restrict decision making to consistently composed teams or to ensure that their members were appropriately trained and provided with careful guidance as to procedure. Arrangements for recording decisions appeared unsystematic in many cases while arrangements for review of all or part of the selection system, and the decisions it produced, were at best uneven. Even in the most systematic example of redesign encountered, no hard data were available in terms of which the effects of the new system on outcomes could be measured.[5]

Finally, we may note that much of the awareness, good practice and innovation revealed by the research was a matter of the initiative of individuals, often working substantially alone. As we shall see in Chapter 6, this feature also characterised examples of good practice in the area of positive action.

## Notes

1 Since our research was completed, the ENB has commissioned a further study based, in part, on the results of our inquiries. It reveals substantially similar patterns, both of application and of success, to those revealed by our work (ENB, 2000).

2 In order to protect the confidentiality and anonymity of individual respondents we refrain, in the discussion that follows, from identifying this institution, even by its pseudonym. We also omit respondent numbers for the same reason.

3 Compare the report of the ENB's Targeted Monitoring of Recruitment for Ethnic Minority Groups for 1998-1999 (ENB 2000: paras. 8.1, 8.2 and 9.1).

4 The ENB's Targeted Monitoring of Recruitment for Ethnic Minority Groups for 1998-1999 (ENB 2000) similarly reported that the area of monitoring and review was the least well advanced of generally weakly developed policy (paras. 7.2-7.3).

5 Our findings here are confirmed by the results of the ENB's subsequent research (ENB 2000). The authors of this study devised an Equal Opportunities Maturity Model, in terms of which institutions providing nursing and midwifery education were rated. They concluded that, on a scale of 0 – 5, the majority of institutions could be said not to have risen above 1. In other words they 'had not progressed significantly beyond a declaration of intent to observe the principle of equal opportunities' (ENB 2000 para. 8.1). Only eighteen per cent of institutions nationally were provisionally awarded a score of 4 and the authors concluded that a more thorough audit might uncover deficiencies not revealed by their preliminary study (para. 8.2).

# 6 Positive Action in Recruitment to Nursing and Midwifery Training

In Chapter 5 we reviewed evidence that, in the majority of institutions studied in our research, good equal opportunities practices were not well embedded in selection systems for nursing and midwifery education. In other words, despite clear evidence of differential success rates among members of different ethnic groups, there was little evidence of any sustained, effective effort to ensure that, in selecting candidates for training, all those applying had a genuinely equal opportunity to be successful. Our results seem to be confirmed by subsequent work by the ENB which concluded that the substantial majority of institutions had not advanced beyond the expression of a generalised statement of intent to observe equal opportunities principles (ENB, 2000: para. 8.1).

It has long been recognised, however, that if equal opportunities policies are to deliver on their objectives, they must extend beyond mere rhetorical commitments to equity and diversity. In addition, there is widespread agreement that equitable arrangements for selecting from among applicants represent only one dimension of the measures necessary to secure genuine equal opportunities. This is because such arrangements, even when well developed and effectively implemented, seeure equity only among those who have been able to enter the competition. They do nothing to address patterns of under-representation among those making applications in the first place. In the context of such arguments, the 1976 Race Relations Act, sections 37-38, made provision for what has become known as 'positive action'. Positive action measures consist of targeted initiatives aimed at increasing the numbers of members of under-represented groups in a workforce. They represent, in other words, one mechanism for translating a formal commitment to equity into a real change in workforce profiles. The 1976 Act focused primarily on unfair discrimination, but it also incorporated a recognition that outlawing discrimination alone would not necessarily alleviate the disadvantage experienced by minority ethnic communities. That recognition was made clear in the U.K. Government's 1975 White Paper *Racial Discrimination* which presented proposals for the Act:

> if the principle of non-discrimination is interpreted too literally and inflexibly it may actually impede the elimination of invidious discrimination and the encouragement of equal opportunity...The Government considers that it would be wrong to adhere so blindly to the principle of formal legal equality as to ignore the handicaps preventing many black and brown workers from obtaining equal employment opportunities (U.K., 1975: para. 57, p.14).

Similarly, the 1974 White Paper, *Equality for Women*, which preceded the 1975 Sex Discrimination Act, stated that:

> An anti-discrimination law is relevant only to the extent that economic and social conditions enable people to develop their individual potential and to compete for opportunities on more or less equal terms (U.K., 1974: para. 21, p.5).

The subsequent Acts were both clear and specific about the positive action measures that could be taken voluntarily by employers. In relation to racial disadvantage, employers are allowed to encourage job applications from members of particular 'racial groups' when there are either no persons of the group employed in a particular area of work at an establishment or when the proportion of the group employed is 'small' in comparison to their proportion amongst all those employed at the establishment or amongst the population of the areas from which an employer normally recruits its workforce (Race Relations Act, 1976: sec. 37-38). Under the same conditions, special training can be provided for members of particular racial groups to help them acquire the skills for particular work. Although there is no legal obligation for employers to make use of the positive action provisions, the Commission for Racial Equality has recommended in its *Code of Practice* (CRE, 1984a: 20) that they are implemented where particular racial groups are under-represented. In essence, the objective of positive action practices was to reduce structural inequalities at work chiefly by helping women and minority ethnic communities to compete on more equitable terms in the workplace. (Preferential treatment, or 'positive discrimination' between individuals at the point of selection for work, is unlawful. All applicants must be considered on merit in relation to job requirements with 'racial' group being a lawful criterion only under very circumscribed conditions.[1])

## Researching Positive Action in the NHS

There is very little research evidence about the extent to which NHS employers have implemented positive action measures. Limited quantitative research suggests that progress has been slow. By 1985 - nine years after positive action was enabled by the 1976 Race Relations Act - only four out of thirty-one London District Health Authorities had established positive action provisions (LACRC, 1985: 29). This increased to five by 1987 (GLARE, 1987: 25). A mail survey of all Health Authorities in the U.K. in 1991, revealed that only 11 per cent of 197 respondent Health Authorities had implemented any positive action measures (Iganski, 1992). More recently, a survey of NHS Trusts in 1993 (EOR, 1994) found that only eight out of 93 had set targets - commonly regarded as an adjunct to positive action initiatives - for the employment of minority ethnic groups.

There is even less qualitative evidence on the operational experience of the establishment of positive action provisions and the factors that enable, or alternatively, impede, such provisions. In the case of health services, research, using case studies in three nurse education centres, indicated a lack of recruitment initiatives targeted at minority ethnic communities, and a lack of ideas for potential initiatives (Gerrish *et al.*, 1996: 118-124). The research discovered some initiatives in the early stages of development but subjected them to little critical scrutiny.

In the remainder of this chapter we report on the outcomes of our investigation of positive action provisions in the eight institutions studied in our research. (We discuss the selection of the institutions, and the selection of respondents, in Chapter 5.) Approximately one-third of our 81 respondents occupied key managerial roles for the recruitment and selection of students, and their accounts inform the material presented in this chapter.

Two broad questions guided our inquiry: to what extent did the institutions specifically target minority ethnic groups in their recruitment activity; and what could be learnt from their activities to provide illustrations for other nurse education centres in particular, and for the establishment of positive action provisions in general?

For the investigation of recruitment measures, we applied a different research style from that used in the investigation of recruitment practices discussed in Chapter 5. We used a grounded theory approach to the collection of data and to the data analysis, although, in a modified form. As is characteristic of a grounded theory approach, we approached data collection and data analysis as dynamic interactive processes, rather than distinct phases of the research. The analysis began formally after the very first interview and even began to develop in the interviewers' minds during the first interview. There was a subsequent constant interaction between data collection and data analysis or, as Bulmer (1984) has termed it, a 'flip-flop' between the emergent ideas and the lines of enquiry pursued in the interviews. This dynamic process is central to a grounded theory approach and means that it is not purely inductive.

No two interviews were the same, therefore, in terms of the questions asked. Ideas that emerged from the ongoing analysis were explored in subsequent interviews. Interviews took the form of 'directed discussions', incorporating elements with varying degrees of structure. For instance in a number of interviews respondents were asked to 'talk through the way students are recruited'. Elsewhere, the researchers drew from an interview checklist that provided the interviewer with a possible agenda of topics for discussion. As already stated, initial coding began in the minds of the interviewers during the interviews. It then continued directly after the interviews in discussions between the researchers in the time-lag between interview and transcription and then proceeded more formally when the transcripts were available. It is in this sense that the approach to data analysis constituted a modified grounded theory approach as we applied initial analyses developed during and after interviews to subsequent interviews, before a full analysis could be carried out on the interview transcript. The tag-lag between interview and transcription necessitated such a strategy.

The use of 'memos' is integral to a grounded theory approach to data analysis. Holloway and Wheeler, in their book; *Qualitative Research for Nurses*, argue that:

> Every grounded theory researcher should write memos. They are meant to help in the development and formulation of theory. In theoretical memos the researcher discusses tentative ideas and provisional categories, compares findings and jots down thoughts on the research. Initially, memos might remind the researcher 'don't forget ... ' or 'I intend to ... '; later they encompass micro-codes, and later still, major emergent categories, hunches, implications and concepts from the literature; memos become more varied and theoretical ... Diagrams in the memos can help to remind the analyst and structure the study ... Eventually, memos become integrated in the writing (1996: 109-110).

The writing of memos for this research project involved an additional modification to the grounded theory approach. Because of the realities of contract research in terms of the constraints on time and resources, the memos were less formalised than Holloway and Wheeler suggest, in that they were written as elements of a draft research report from a very early stage in the analytic process. As the ideas and theory developed, and the memos correspondingly developed, the research report was drafted and re-drafted, and began to take shape. The memos therefore constituted the elements of a countless number of draft reports.

## Positive Action in Recruitment to Nurse Education

The research found mixed progress in terms of the establishment of positive action provisions. Two of the centres carried out no specific targeting of minority ethnic communities in their recruitment activities and there was considerable variation in practice among the remaining six centres. Moreover, the interview data indicated that there were three key areas in which this variability could be detected. These were: the availability/acceptance of a *rationale* for action; the availability of *information* (in particular, data on the ethnic composition of student populations and the local labour force); and the existence of a *strategy* for action. We suggest, in line with much of the policy literature, that an effective *system* for the implementation of positive action provisions entails the development and integration of these three elements. In other words, effective positive action implies not simply an acceptance of the arguments for such action but also the availability of information in terms of which to develop initiatives and the formulation of an action plan in terms of which to act and evaluate progress (cf. CRE, 1989; U.K. Employment Department, 1991). Yet, as we shall see, each of these elements was variably underdeveloped in the institutions studied while in no case was a feedback loop closed between the three elements (cf. CRE, 1989). In the final section of the paper we identify some of the reasons for this limited and uneven progress. First, however, we present evidence from our case studies in relation to each of the three elements identified above.

*A Rationale for Positive Action*

In general, more active measures were taken to target potential applicants from minority ethnic communities in those institutions where pragmatic arguments for doing so were most strongly articulated. The force of such arguments was not, however, recognised in all of the centres. In the Saltash Institute of Health, for instance, the Academic Coordinator - responsible for some recruitment initiatives - noted that although the organisation aimed to recruit from the local population, there was no specific targeting of minority ethnic groups:

> We never look for a shortage of ethnic minorities, we look for a shortage of students (011).

This comment indicates how some respondents adopted what might be described as a 'colour-blind' approach to recruitment. For instance, the Academic Coordinator at Saltash felt it was not necessary to target minority ethnic groups within the local population in order to attract them into training, since localised recruitment would inevitably draw from these groups:

> I don't think there is a conscious effort to recruit one or the other, it's that the local population is made up in this manner therefore workers are going to be because they happen to be living here ... if you go to the North Sea you fish cod, what you get is cod, if you go to the Portuguese ... coast you're going to get sardines (011).

A recruitment team leader at the Peverell Institute of Health made a similar point:

> I must say that it's normal here ... the ethnic community is so much part of the local community ... we don't target them because we don't see them as any different to be honest (019).

Neither of these managers appeared to be aware of, or to accept, the arguments for specifically targeting minority ethnic groups. A lecturer involved in recruitment events at the Eggbuckland Institute of Health reported that a conscious decision had been made not to target recruitment activities and expressed a feeling of unease about doing so on the grounds that it might imply discrimination:

> I would like to say ... that I don't actively target anybody or actively discourage anybody, I would like to think that we attend schools and other promotional functions in as value free a manner as is possible for any human being to do and if anyone comes up and says 'tell me about nursing', you tell them about nursing and personally I think I would be as uncomfortable with targeting groups of people as the thought that someone was disadvantaged for a reason other than they weren't suited to it (048).

This statement implies that positive action is seen as a form of preferential treatment, or positive discrimination. Such a confusion of positive action with positive discrimination has been evident in other research (Jewson *et al.*, 1990; Moore, 1997: 116) and has arguably served as a significant barrier to the establishment of positive action (Rubenstein, 1986).

Other respondents, however, did offer some pragmatic arguments for positive action. First the connection between the recruitment of minority ethnic students and the provision of health care sensitive to the needs of minority ethnic communities was articulated by some respondents. For instance, a senior administrator responsible for recruitment at Mannamead observed that:

> Quite simply we need more people from ethnic minorities in the health service and in particular I think in nursing ... we've got a high ethnic minority population here and I'm not just talking about Asians, I'm talking about people from African backgrounds as well, all minority groups. It's important that we have a workforce that's going to reflect the people that we're caring for. Plus, it's a slow process, it's not just us you see, you've got the police force in the area that have initiatives, the armed forces nationally have got initiatives, so I think everybody's trying to get a more representative workforce and it's who can show themselves to be more attractive (003).

A senior nurse manager within the Lipson Institute of Health also offered a very clear rationale for recruiting students from local minority ethnic communities:

> ... we feel very committed to trying to provide nurses from the same ethnic background as our community ... I am not saying that in order to get the best nursing care you've got to be nursed by somebody from your own culture, I think that would be absurd and would be insulting people, but I think to know that within the team that's caring for you, that there is somebody who will understand, not just interaction with you but will also plan your care taking into account that for instance you might not want to be examined by a male doctor, there is somebody in that team who will be attuned to those kind of issues (023).

However, such a need for positive action was not articulated by all managers responsible for recruitment, indicating perhaps that national policy exhortation has not permeated all education centres, even at the most senior levels. Alternatively, it may also indicate that needs recognised by those involved in day to day service delivery have not been articulated in ways which have reached those responsible for recruitment to the profession.[2]

Interviews with other senior managers responsible for recruitment suggested a further rationale for targeted recruitment initiatives, although it was used to justify localised recruitment in general rather than the specific targeting of minority ethnic communities. Some managers reported that they were under pressure from health service providers who contracted their training places to recruit locally in order to achieve a stable nursing workforce and reduce staff turnover. For instance, the Contracts Manager for the Wembury Institute of Health - which recruits some students from Ireland - stated that:

> ... because we've had difficulties recruiting here we've been recruiting in Ireland … considerable numbers … I think there's a concern that recruiting people in Ireland isn't actually going to ... at the end of the day ... perhaps enhance the local workforce because people might go back or elsewhere. Whereas if you recruit locally those people are likely to stay and work locally afterwards, which is obviously the main concern (035).

It was clear from the Contracts Manager's further comments that the concern was chiefly about recruiting a stable workforce:

> The main pressure I think is to recruit locally and not recruit from Ireland … a few people applying and coming through the system, fine … but not having major recruitment drives in Ireland … you know there's concern I think about having a large number of people from one place who haven't got any loyalty or connection with the area that they're training in and therefore may not then be going back into the local workforce (035).

An Administration Manager from the Saltash Institute of Health Studies, which also recruits from Ireland, provided an almost identical rationale for focusing recruitment on the local population:

> If you encourage more people from the local community you get a better cross section of people from all ethnic backgrounds ... in addition it would make sense to encourage people from local communities because once they've qualified they are more likely to

> take up permanent work within the local hospitals, whereas for instance although students from Ireland are keen to come here, a lot of them will eventually want to go back to Ireland to do their nursing once they qualify (007).

This argument for localised recruitment provided a pragmatic rationale for positive action measures which had been recognised in at least one of the education centres. If minority ethnic communities are targeted in the localities in which education centres are based there is the potential dual advantage of recruiting students who will be more likely to remain with local health providers once they qualify, and at the same time, increasing the ethnic diversity of the local nursing workforce.

A third pragmatic justification lies in the labour supply potential of Britain's minority ethnic groups. The black and Asian communities in Britain represent a significant pool of potential young workers as the age profile of the groups is younger in comparison with the population as a whole. In the 1991 population Census one-third of the ethnic minorities as a whole were aged under 16 compared with just under one fifth of the white population. Whilst the minority ethnic groups accounted for 5.49 per cent of the population overall, they accounted for a larger proportion (9.04 per cent) of under 16-year-olds (U.K. Office of Population Censuses and Surveys, 1993).

A senior academic at the Mannamead Institute of Health clearly recognised the labour supply potential of minority ethnic communities:

> ... there's also the sheer question of numbers. We have a very large immigrant population here. Recruitment of nurses for the future: we have to - in terms of numbers - get people in, there will be insufficient people who provide care (015).

However, this was the only respondent who provided an argument for positive action in these terms. Of all the eight nurse education and training institutions studied, the Mannamead Institute of Health is located in an area where the minority ethnic communities constitute the highest proportion of the local population. The importance of these communities as a source of labour was, therefore, perhaps felt the most acutely there. However, all of the other institutions are located in areas where the percentage of minority ethnic groups as a proportion of the local population is higher than the figure for England as a whole. The omission by the remaining senior managers responsible for recruitment is therefore surprising. It is perhaps even more surprising in view of the efforts of the Department of Health to make health service employers aware of the labour supply potential of the minority ethnic groups. However, it is perhaps more readily understood when it is appreciated that few of the senior managers responsible for recruitment knew the ethnic group composition of their localities or of their cohorts of students and were, therefore, unable to make informed comparisons.

*Information: Applicant Monitoring Data*

Most equal opportunity recommendations emphasise the importance of data collection on the ethnic group composition of job applicants and the monitoring of the outcome of applications by ethnic group (see, for example, CRE, 1989; U.K. Employment Department, 1991; Jewson *et al.*, 1992). Monitoring data may provide *prima facie* evidence of unlawful discrimination if they reveal differential selection outcomes for applicants from different ethnic groups - a pattern which can then be subject to further investigation. More generally, data on applicants will also indicate whether they are representative of the recruitment pool from which they are drawn and whether positive action provisions may be necessary and legally justifiable in terms of the provisions of the 1976 Race Relations Act. In this context, then, data on the representation of minority ethnic groups amongst applicants to training for nursing provides an essential pre-requisite for targeted recruitment initiatives. Institutions require data on the ethnic group composition of applicants and recruits, the ethnic group composition of the locality from which they recruit and, the ethnic group composition of the populations likely to be served by the recruits once trained. There is, of course, a national and international recruitment pool for training in nursing and midwifery and there is no guarantee that recruits once qualified will remain in the localities in which they have been trained. Nevertheless, the populations proximate to the education centres and the health care providers to which they are contracted provide the best approximations of the populations against which the ethnic group composition of applicants can be compared. Moreover, as we have seen, some recruiters themselves recognised a tendency for locally recruited staff subsequently to work in the locality.

Statistical data on applicants to training in nursing and midwifery were provided to education centres by the Nurses and Midwives Central Clearing House (NMCCH) in the early 1990s. However, in 1993 problems with a new database system interrupted data provision. In September 1997 the Nursing and Midwifery Admissions Service (NMAS) succeeded the NMCCH in administering applications. It is contracted to provide data to centres on a quarterly basis, and at the end of each fixed application period, on applicants by ethnic group, sex, age group, educational qualifications and application outcome. These data will be incomplete, however, as they will not include information on applicants applying directly to institutions and who do not register their applications with NMAS. All the eight case study centres accepted direct applications at the time of the research and such applications will still be permitted under the new system. Since for some institutions the proportions of direct applicants are large, the omissions in the data may be considerable. Amongst the case study institutions the proportions of direct applicants ranged from 5 per cent at the Lipson Institute to an estimated forty-five per cent at the Wembury Institute. The proportion of direct applicants had reached seventy per cent on one occasion at the Keyham Institute.

In this context then, we were interested in whether the eight education centres had established their own applicant monitoring systems during the four-year period in which the NMCCH data were interrupted, whether they had initiated monitoring of direct applicants which would be needed to supplement the data provided by NMAS, and whether measures had been established to use monitoring data to inform recruitment initiatives; including seeking population data by ethnic group for their localities.

Interviews with responsible senior managers, and others involved in recruitment processes, revealed a great deal of uncertainty about whether applicant monitoring data were available and, perhaps more significantly, about the potential use of such data. Overall, although some institutions appeared to collect relevant information, none used ethnic group data on applicants to inform their recruitment strategies. This was the case even for those institutions that had established some positive action initiatives. This itself is a matter of some interest since positive action is technically only lawful in the context of an evident under-representation of the targeted group. In addition, none of the respondents appeared to be aware of the availability of Census[3] or other population data for the localities from which they recruited and which might serve to indicate whether there was under- or over-representation of particular groups amongst applicants.

A few examples from the case study centres serve to illustrate these observations. At the Saltash Institute of Health, there was a notable lack of consensus between respondents about the representation of minority ethnic groups amongst applicants and about how they compared to the local population. The staff interviewed reported that they had not seen regular reports on the ethnic composition of either applications to training, or student cohorts. For example, the Academic Coordinator justified the absence of targeting on his perception of the representation of minority ethnic groups at the Institute's graduation ceremonies:

> ... we've got an awards ceremony and see who comes to get the awards, and we are well represented, there is no doubt in that (011).

By contrast, a recruitment administrator at Saltash justified holding open days targeted at local minority ethnic communities on the basis of 'a feeling' (022) that they were not getting enough pre-registration training applications from those communities. A lecturer expressed the belief that data were kept on the ethnic group profile of students - but not applicants - but had experienced difficulty in accessing the data when it had been requested (030). The heads of the Nursing and Midwifery branches at Saltash reported that they did not know whether the Institute held data on applications. Whilst they expressed the belief that ethnic group data on students were recorded they had not seen any reports and did not, therefore, know whether the data were analysed or used in any way.

There was a similar situation at the Keyham Institute. The senior administrator responsible for recruitment explained:

> We do keep statistical information ... yearly from the direct applications, and from the applicants that come through the Nurses and Midwives Central Clearing House ... we do statistical information about the ethnic origin, their age, male and female ... and also the ones that we've interviewed and how many we actually accepted, we do a breakdown of that statistical information as well ... basically the

> information I compile … yearly, so it's there available if anyone requires it …
>
> Q. Is the information used to feed into the marketing … ?
>
> I don't think it is … basically we compile it and we look at it because if we didn't do it someone would then come and ask us for it, so we do it automatically so it's there if anybody wants it … (081).

A senior administrator at the Eggbuckland Institute who was responsible for planning the development of the database systems clearly could not see how ethnic group data could be used in recruitment, and confused lawful positive action measures with unlawful positive discrimination:

> We're not into positive discrimination and I suppose if we were and the decision was made that you should be doing that sort of thing then we could use the data but I mean that's not what it's there for ... I mean it's a difficult thing, we've got nothing to compare to really and so you can't say oh well, we're generally doing okay or we're not, then you are operating in a vacuum.

*Targeting Strategy*

It was clear from the case studies of the eight nurse education centres that some managers responsible for the recruitment of students had few ideas about how to target potential applicants from minority ethnic communities. For instance, the Academic Coordinator at the Wembury Institute explained:

> ... we don't prepare materials specifically for Asian groups ... I don't know how one would do that really...all our material is in English, but then it's necessary to do that in that you would expect people coming in to, you know, be able to speak English ... I'm not quite sure about how we would target those groups more finely than by targeting organisations like schools and colleges where the local ethnic make-up is reflected in those organisations ... you know, unless one targeted the local temple or mosque or whatever (laughter) (035).

The senior administrator for the South Wembury sites clearly saw the need for positive action measures but, again, could offer few ideas about how recruitment could be targeted:

> When I go to careers evenings in the schools I try to focus to the parents ... you know the student might say 'I wish to do nursing' and the parents say 'No, no, no, no', you know, and I try and talk to them, talk through it with them and they're getting better, but we haven't actually sat down and worked out how to go through it maybe in the community as such (034).

However, various positive action measures were taken by some of the institutions studied and the interviews with senior managers suggested that, to be effective, positive action initiatives need to constitute an adequately resourced strategy of action rather than simply *ad hoc*, poorly resourced, interventions. It was also evident that regularly used recruitment channels could be adapted to targeting potential students from minority ethnic communities. Both of these observations can be illustrated by interview data.

First, given the concerns expressed by respondents about the attractiveness of nursing to members of some minority groups, one measure that institutions might take to attract applicants would be to establish links with minority ethnic community organisations to clarify and promote career opportunities. Whilst youth and young adult groups would provide pools of potential applicants, links might also be established with other community groups. For instance, parents could also provide a channel for encouragement and might, in some cases, themselves need to have their concerns allayed. Three of the case study centres had established such links.

At the Mannamead Institute of Health the senior administrator responsible for recruitment is invited occasionally through informal contacts to speak to groups about careers in nursing. She had also established regular links with one particular group on her own initiative. She explained her activities not simply as targeting the group for recruitment purposes but in terms of a concern with raising the profile of the Institute within the community and generally encouraging the idea of a career in nursing:

> There's a group that I go and meet with and they are women who have either not been in this country very long or they may have been in this country but their language skills are not very good and some of them have degrees from Pakistan so really at the moment it's a bit of a sort of PR exercise and a social exercise in that I go and meet with them and you think to yourself there's so much talent there, once they've got the language skills that they'll cope with the course hopefully, we would encourage them (003).

However, this respondent was acting on her own initiative in developing such links and they were neither formally resourced as part of her regular responsibilities, nor part of a formalised recruitment strategy. In the Peverell Institute of Health, a recruitment team leader explained that contact had been made with groups from two different ethnic minority communities to which talks on nursing had been given (021). However, this initiative had been terminated because it was not believed to have increased the number of minority ethnic applicants:

> ... we haven't done that for about 18 months because even that didn't really work. At the end of the day you could see no significant increase in ethnic minority candidates coming forward (021).

It is difficult to evaluate the efforts of single individuals in trying to increase the number of applications from minority ethnic groups and it is not surprising that this initiative was difficult to sustain. As the respondent pointed out, there needs to be a more strategic, and properly resourced, approach to links with communities in order to evaluate their effectiveness as recruitment activities:

> ... it's not for me to say whether the images we portray connect with any grouping, we'd have to go out and do some fieldwork and find out ... we do need to make some more formal contacts with...the leaders of the ethnic communities (025).

The Lipson Institute of Health provides an example of a possible model for establishing links with minority ethnic community groups. The Institute has employed a recruitment officer specifically to engage in outreach work with some of the local communities. As a senior nurse manager explained:

> ... we have at the moment a point five [0.5] recruitment officer who goes into schools and she's been doing some particular work with three communities in the main (023).

The manager felt that outreach work of this nature involved breaking down barriers to entry into nursing and altering attitudes. Both required a sustained, long-term, commitment:

> ... it needs a lot of going back time and time again reiterating maybe the same message but in different ways, to help the local community understand that this is their university and their school, you know, and not to be afraid to come forward or to break down the prejudices in relation to nursing ... and alerting us to things ... to identify things we hadn't thought of (023).

All of the eight case study centres provided careers information and advice in schools and colleges. One of the institutions specifically targeted minority ethnic groups in this way. The Mannamead Institute had established, in collaboration with the local Training and Enterprise Council, a 'mentor scheme' with a school with a high proportion of minority ethnic students. Despite its good intentions, however, there are clearly resource limitations to the scheme. It is organised mostly by one person - the senior administrator responsible for recruitment - with voluntary contributions from the teaching staff but with no mentors from minority ethnic groups:

> We've set up an arrangement now with one of the schools in the area which is 95 per cent ethnic minority and they've set up a mentoring scheme, so we've got several members of the ... teaching staff and myself, we are going in to mentor groups and individual students ... The people who have, I would say volunteered to go, who have got the time to go at the moment, no they're not ... staff who are from ethnic minorities ... It isn't that they're not interested, at the moment they couldn't meet the commitment (003).

Another centre, the Saltash Institute of Health, operated a scheme which could potentially be used to target minority ethnic groups, although it was not explicitly used for that purpose. In order to promote training opportunities the Academic Coordinator at the Institute had negotiated what were described as 'contracts' with some local colleges of further education for students undertaking access courses. The Institute had contracted to guarantee an interview to all access students who passed their courses and applied for training. Anecdotal evidence was provided from other institutions that there are high proportions of minority ethnic students undertaking access courses as a route into higher and further education. This initiative, therefore, could be seen as a way to attract minority ethnic groups into training. However, this was clearly not seen as the primary purpose of the scheme.

> I think [this] is going to pay very good dividends because the people are mature, these people have gone to a lot of trouble to do those courses and they will be very good stayers in the programme so the wastage would be much less and they will be local people, they don't need residency and things like that so I think we're on a winner (011).

It is sometimes argued that positive role models can be helpful in attracting applicants for positions in which members of particular groups have traditionally been absent, excluded or under-represented. In this context, a number of respondents in four of the eight education centres had consciously tried to involve students and staff from minority ethnic groups in recruitment activities. One tutor from the Eggbuckland Institute of Health had involved a Black student in a recruitment event at a local school:

> I quite deliberately took a black female student with me to one of them ... I said because you are a black woman and I want you to come along and be seen to be there, and talk by all means honestly and openly about your experience ... I do think that she could have a positive influence on the recruitment of black people, better than I can. She could answer their questions openly and honestly if they did have any sensitive questions they wanted to ask her (045).

'Role models' were similarly used in the Wembury Institute of Health in careers visits to schools but the arrangements were very *ad hoc*:

> If we can get students to come with us we do ... but their timetables and commitments, you know, they sometimes can't always fit us in ... we have got, if you like, some tutors that would relate to this particular area, and we take them along to see if it will help relieve the problem (034).

The Devonport Institute of Health also had very *ad hoc* arrangements. The Administration Manager pointed out what she believed were some of the constraints involved:

> ... when we go to careers conventions we try to get a mix of staff on the careers stands, but that's often easier said than done and it's down to who's available and so on ... I think it's probably a resource matter ... this working group on equal opportunities, one of the people on it ... feels very very strongly about it that we should be doing more than we do, one of the things for instance that she suggested in a particular area of Devonport ... (is that) ... when we go into that school ... identifying a qualified nurse who speaks, from the same background, who speaks the same language. Now, ideally yes, I can see that but the logistics of trying to organise that, to try and have that sort of detailed information to try and make contact with that sort of person in the hospital and then get them to come to the event with us is really not realistic (004).

There appears to be a clear rationale for using 'role models' - both staff and students - in careers events designed to attract potential applicants from minority ethnic groups and some respondents clearly felt that they could perform a valuable role. Others, however, had understandable reservations. For some the concern was that the notion of 'role models' might imply a labelling of the minority ethnic staff involved. For others, the issue was one of the demands on the limited time of the usually small number of senior staff available to act in these capacities. The experiences of the education centres reveal the limitations of relying on volunteers to act without recompense for their efforts. It would appear that if this strategy is to be effective, and if staff from minority ethnic groups are to be encouraged to attend it needs to be part of the designated responsibilities of staff and not dependent just upon goodwill.

## Conclusion

We have seen, then, that in the eight nurse education centres studied few positive action provisions had been established which were adequately resourced, part of a systematic strategy of targeting minority ethnic communities, or informed by data on those communities and on the characteristics of applicants and student cohorts. Most of the measures encountered were inappropriately resourced and *ad hoc* and commonly relied on the initiative of particularly committed individuals. Given the relatively strong rhetorical national commitments to greater representativeness in the NHS workforce, and the fact that the eight centres were located in areas which might reasonably have been expected to facilitate effective targeting of minority ethnic groups, we may pose the question: 'Why were so few effective initiatives in place?'

We suggested above that there were three key elements in terms of which linked progress required to be made before effective positive action measures could be expected. These were: the availability/acceptance of a *rationale* for action, the availability of *information* about the ethnic composition of student populations and the local labour force, and the existence of a *strategy* for action. Our evidence shows that all three of these elements were under-developed to varying degrees in the centres studied and that there was little systematic linkage between the three such that a feedback loop could be established on the basis of which to review and further develop action plans.

It was evident that where a rationale for positive action was most clearly articulated the most developed initiatives were to be found. This is, perhaps, not surprising since acceptance of a rationale typically precedes decisions to act.[4] What is most noteworthy in this context, therefore, is the fact that the various available arguments and rationales were neither fully and widely understood nor wholeheartedly embraced. This suggests that the message of national policy commitments and their rationale, as discussed in Chapter 3 of this book, had not been efficiently disseminated, and that arrangements for communication, education and training - particularly of those staff involved in recruitment and selection - were less than effective. It may also be the case, however, that there are more significant limitations in the kinds of arguments characteristically used to justify equal opportunities measures. In the final two chapters, we consider some of these issues and place them in the context of more general questions concerning both the nature of equal opportunities and the increasingly diverse character of Britain's multi-ethnicity.

## Notes

1 Edwards has questioned whether this distinction can, in practice, be easily upheld (1995).

2 Other research, however, suggests that sensitivity to the implications of ethnic diversity for health care provision is not necessarily widespread among the nursing and midwifery workforce (Bowler, 1993).

3 Census data are not without their problems of course. There may be no clear overlap between the localities served, or recruited from, by a given institution and the geographical units in respect of which Census data are available. More importantly, there are a number of specific difficulties with ethnic data derived from the Census. These include the partial coverage and fuzziness of the Census categories and the differential under-enumeration of different ethnic groups. (See the discussion in Bulmer, 1996.) Having said that, the key issue here is the lack of awareness of the availability even of imperfect data and its implications for policy development.

4 Although, of course, we should note that people sometimes act under duress or instruction without embracing the underlying rationale.

# 7 Social Change and the Health Care Agenda

Thus far we have noted that the NHS has experienced a range of difficulties in responding adequately to the unfolding equality agenda. These difficulties have ranged from those associated with a failure to grasp the nettle of inequity and racism, to those which have their origins in organisational structures that frustrate attempts to translate emergent national commitments into effective action 'on the ground'. The analysis in Chapter 6 illustrated how the fragmented organisational structure of the NHS had direct implications both for the dissemination of good practice, and for the monitoring and review of progress. There is reason to believe, however, that the issues that need to be addressed, if effective progress towards greater equity is to be achieved, are not confined to questions either of commitment or organisation.

We may usefully take the discussion in Chapter 6 about one aspect of local practice as a way into a more sophisticated understanding of the challenges facing the NHS and, by extension, the attempt to secure equity and full substantive citizenship more generally in British national life.

As we saw, there was a good deal of uncertainty among our respondents in nursing and midwifery education centres about the kinds and appropriateness of ethnic monitoring data available to them. There was even less clarity about the kinds of data available regarding the ethnic makeup of local labour markets or of the recruitment pool, in terms of which the success or otherwise of targeted recruitment initiatives might effectively be judged. Some of these uncertainties can clearly be explained in terms of the lack of awareness of staff and, by extension, the weaknesses in arrangements for training and dissemination of good practice. Others, however, seem to relate more directly to a failure of the available data to have been analysed and presented in a manner that permitted direct comparisons between the application and selection profile of institutions and the localities from which they recruited. Indeed, there seemed to be little evidence that most respondents had any sophisticated understanding of the ethnic makeup of their recruitment pools and even less knowledge of the cultures and traditions of the groups concerned. Partly as a result, respondents were all too ready to invoke stereotyped characterisations of other cultures as explanations for their failure to attract applicants from particular groups.

Clearly, there are some basic practical issues here which might be resolved, given the will, by more sophisticated interrogation of Census and personnel data and by more effective training. There are, however, reasons to believe that there are some more complex conceptual issues about the nature of ethnic difference, and the means by which it is measured, that impact directly on policy implementation and on the framing of arguments for greater equity. These issues are further complicated by processes of social change which, there is reason to believe, may be outpacing some conventional and taken for granted understandings of the character of ethnic diversity in modern Britain.

## Ethnic Difference as a Problem

In Britain, both in popular parlance and the framing of social policy, ethnic difference is almost exclusively associated with an implicit division of the population into an ethnic 'majority' and a number of ethnic minorities. This distinctive British perspective is substantially a product of the pattern of migration to Britain since the Second World War, a period which has seen the growth of a population whose recent origins lie in the former British colonies in the Indian subcontinent, the Caribbean, Africa, and the so-called Far East. Initially designated in both official and popular parlance as 'immigrants', this population has increasingly become known as 'ethnic minorities'. Two points about this terminology are significant.

The first is that in order to qualify for designation as an ethnic minority, a category of people must exhibit a degree of 'difference' that is regarded as significant. As a result, not every group having a distinctive culture and constituting a minority in the British population is normally included. Thus, the large communities of people of Cypriot, Italian and Polish origin (to name only a few) to be found in many British cities are rarely thought of as constituting ethnic minorities. Similarly, people of Irish descent, a significant proportion of the British population (Mason, 2000: 21) are rarely so designated. In practice, it is an unstable combination of skin colour and culture that marks off 'ethnic minorities' from the 'majority' population in Britain. The second point is that, despite the implicit emphasis on difference, 'ethnic minorities' are typically seen to have more in common with one another than with the 'majority'. *Diversity among* the groups so designated is thus downplayed while their purported *differences from* the rest of the population are exaggerated.

It is important to stress that this is not necessarily a conscious process. Nor is it driven simply by those committed to explicitly racist, or otherwise exclusionary, political projects – such as far right political parties. Even initiatives driven by a commitment to policies designed to address ethnic disadvantage and exclusion find it difficult to escape these assumptions. An example is the 1991 Census of Population which included a question designed to measure the ethnic diversity of the British population and map differences of experience and opportunity (Coleman and Salt, 1996: 9-10). For the first time all members of the population were asked to identify their ethnic group. Even a brief perusal of the relevant question on the Census form illustrates the key point at issue.

Respondents were invited to chose from among the following categories:

White
Black—Caribbean
Black—African
Black—Other (please describe)
Indian
Pakistani
Bangladeshi
Chinese
Any other ethnic group (please describe)

Thus those who ticked 'White' were not required further to differentiate themselves. It is difficult to escape the conclusion either that 'White' was regarded as a unitary identity or that differences within it were seen as of little importance. At the same time, the other categories offered represent a curious mishmash of principles of differentiation. Thus they mix, in a variety of inconsistent ways, skin colour, geographical origin, and nationality or citizenship categories. In practice, the only thing that unites them is that they are all presumed to capture the ethnic identities of those members of the population whose skin-colour is thought of as not being white. Thus the apparent recognition of diversity is immediately undermined by their definition, in practice, by exclusion – they are not white.[1]

A further dimension of this problem is the distinctive character of British conceptions of ethnicity itself (see the fuller discussion in Mason, 2000: 13-14). Characteristically, the term 'ethnic' is taken to refer only to those who are thought of as different from some presumed norm and is frequently used as a synonym for those thought of as culturally different. Talk of an ethnic 'look' in the world of fashion, or of ethnic cuisine, are only two, relatively trivial, examples of the way white British people are apt to see ethnicity as an attribute only of others – something that distinguishes 'them' from 'us'. Moreover, this apparent denial of their own ethnicity also seems to be associated with a distinctively individualistic world-view. '"We" are individuals, "they" are members of groups.' The greater the degree of apparent difference between themselves and others, the more likely British people are to see 'groupishness' as a characteristic of the behaviour and motivations of those others (Dhooge, 1981). One implication of this, in an employment context, is that a failure to attract applicants from groups conceptualised in this way can all too easily be attributed to the characteristics of the groups concerned, rather than to the operation of exclusionary processes, or to the rational decision-making of individuals. The invoking of parental pressure, or supposed cultural prohibitions or preferences, by some of the respondents in our research may well represent examples of this process at work.

A subtext of this kind of thinking is that 'ethnic minorities' themselves constitute a problem. In the context of this discussion they are a problem because they apparently fail to respond to invitations to join the ranks of the nursing and midwifery professions. This parallels processes in other institutions in which they are under-represented, but which have set themselves the goals of recruiting them. Examples include the police and the armed services (see the discussion in Dandeker and Mason, 2001). As one of the authors has been told by senior military personnel, 'Our *problem* is that they won't apply. We need to identify and overcome the barriers that exist in ethnic minority communities to joining the armed services' (private conversation).

This identification of minority ethnic communities as a problem for health service recruiters represents only the latest in a long list of respects in which minority ethnic groups have been seen to present a problem for the health service, or to be the authors of their own misfortunes. All of them are linked to the assimilationist assumptions which have long underpinned health policy and practice (Mason, 2000). They have manifested themselves in a variety of guises, including attacks on traditional health practices, the supposedly deleterious health consequences of the 'Asian' diet, scares about tuberculosis, and the relative lack of attention paid to illnesses specific to minority ethnic groups such as sickle cell disease and thalassaemia. (See the discussions in Ahmad, 1992; 1993; Donovan, 1986; McNaught, 1988; Mason, 2000.)

Three enduring themes, then, have run through British conceptions of ethnicity and, by extension, through social policy – not least in the field of health. The first is that ethnic difference is framed, ultimately by a distinction between a majority (known variously as 'the indigenous population', 'the host society' and the 'white population') and a minority population (characteristically referred to as 'the ethnic minority population' or, in more sophisticated plural variants, 'ethnic minority communities'). This distinction is marked ultimately, and whatever circumlocutions are employed, by differences of skin colour, captured in the end by a distinction between 'white' and 'black' or 'non-white'. The second theme, evident at least from the onset of large scale, post-war, migration to Britain from the countries of the former British Empire, is that the presence of this minority population represents a problem.[2] Typically, minority ethnic groups have been represented as *constituting* a problem. They were, and remain, a problem for those white people who object to their very presence. They were a problem for Governments and others charged with meeting the needs of newly arrived migrants lacking key cultural resources – such as English language skills. They have from time to time been represented as the sources of problems such as certain kinds of street crime or health risks. Most recently, as we have seen, they have been seen as a problem because they appear unwilling to respond positively to attempt to recruit them to key national institutions, including the nursing workforce.

The third theme, follows in many ways from the first. This is that, increasingly sophisticated attempts to disaggregate the minority population notwithstanding, there is a tendency to conceptualise this population as relatively unchanging both in terms of its boundaries and in terms of the problems to which it is thought to be victim. Thus even among those sensitive to equality issues, there is a tendency to assume that the problem is to address more sensitively the employment and other needs of categories of people currently recognised as excluded. Those categories, however, are to some degree ossified by the very methods used to identify the patterning of those needs; notably in the Census and other ethnic monitoring categories. The problem, however, is that any such system must always be working with historical data – a problem which is compounded when the categories used for measurement are rooted in historically conceived problems, framed by the gross conceptual distinction between a 'white' majority and 'black' or 'brown' minorities. In other words, it is particularly ill-attuned to keeping pace with changes in the experiences and, crucially, self-identities of those thought to be members of the categories concerned.

The result is that even those most alive to equality issues are frequently forced to work with categories that are constantly being overtaken by events. We may explore this issue further by looking briefly at recent evidence on social mobility and identities.[3]

## Occupational, Educational and Social Mobility

It has until recently been commonplace to assume that the labour market experience of members of minority ethnic groups has been universally one of disadvantage and exclusion. Without in any way minimising the weight of evidence that points in this direction (see the discussion in Mason, 2000), it is important to note the complexity of the ways in which the rapid economic change of the 1980s and early 1990s has affected existing patterns of advantage and disadvantage in the labour market. An increasing number of studies in the early 1990s (Jones, 1993; Modood, 1997a) had already begun to suggest that members of some groups were experiencing significant upward occupational mobility. The growth of a middle class of professional and managerial workers in some ethnic communities, and the entry of these groups into the service sector, has led some to suggest that there is underway a convergence in the class structures of minority ethnic groups towards that of the white population (Iganski and Payne, 1996;

1999). These trends have been confirmed by the most recent analyses of data for the late 1990s. These suggest that, in terms of economic activity, unemployment and job levels, even some of the previously most disadvantaged groups, Pakistanis and Bangladeshis, have continued to close the gap with whites (Iganski, Payne and Roberts, 2000).

We should note that the patterns are complex, particularly in relation to differences between men and women, and we should avoid jumping to too many conclusions about future patterns of minority ethnic disadvantage.[4] There remain significant differences between members of different ethnic groups, with those of Caribbean descent in particular apparently still lagging behind. Moreover, there are marked regional variations with significant local pockets of labour market disadvantage and exclusion affecting even those groups apparently experiencing upward mobility. Indeed patterns of exclusion altogether from the labour market must be taken into account when considering the successes of those in work. The same is true for the differences between the experiences of women and men. We should also remember that upward mobility is not incompatible with occupational segregation, or with continuing discrimination. We know, for example, that there may be important differences of level *within* broad occupational categories, such as those between senior and middle management. Indeed, these have historically been of great significance in the nursing profession, with minority ethnic nurses having been markedly over-represented among lower status, State Enrolled Nurses (Ward 1993).

What this evidence does point to, however, is a need to place any discussion of the attractiveness to potential minority ethnic recruits of a career in nursing (or, indeed, other hard to recruit to occupations) in the context of a recognition that the range of other opportunities open to them is also changing. The evidence about educational attainment further reinforces this point.

It is clear that members of minority ethnic groups are more likely to remain in full-time education after the age of 16 than are their white counterparts - a finding which holds both for young men and young women (Modood, 1997b). Moreover, the evidence suggests that this is a pattern of relatively longstanding, dating back at least to the beginning of the 1980s (Brown, 1984; U.K. Department of Education and Science, 1985; Drew *et al.*, 1992; Jones, 1993). In addition, it appears that, in general, minority ethnic groups are over-represented in higher education relative to their presence in the population as a whole, although this gross observation conceals some important variations (Jones, 1993: 32; Modood, 1997b; Modood and Ackland, 1998; Modood and Shiner, 1994).

There are a number of potential explanations for this pattern of post-16 educational participation (see the discussion in Mason, 2000). However, Modood (1998) has argued that it is important not to under-estimate the strength of what he calls 'ethnic minorities' drive for qualifications'. He attributes this to a strong motivation for economic betterment in which education is seen to play a key part. In addition, he suggests that qualifications are seen as a means to circumvent persistent labour market discrimination.

The results of the fourth PSI survey concerning qualification levels add further to this picture of progress. Although the patterns are complex (see the discussion in Mason, 2000), they appear to confirm Modood's observations about the progress made by minority ethnic groups relative to whites. Minority ethnic young women, in particular, have made great strides in educational attainment over a relatively short time span. Once again, any analysis of the likely attractiveness of a nursing career must be placed in this context.

## Changing Ethnic Identities

The evidence about occupational and social mobility suggests that conventional categories underplay ethnic diversity both in terms of range and the patterning of change in experience. Equally significantly, they also fail to capture in any precise way, the subtleties of individual and collective identities. Despite considerable pre-testing, it is evident that the 1991 Census question failed fully to capture the self-chosen identities of many of Britain's minority ethnic citizens, resulting in a need for considerable interpretation at the coding stage (see the discussion in Coleman and Salt, 1996). This was one of the reasons for the revisions introduced into the 2001 Census question. Nevertheless, it is doubtful that these changes have fully resolved the problem. One reason is that the Census is constrained to use categories that map in some way onto the patterns believed to underlie the social problems to which solutions are sought (see the discussion above). Any such system of categories is bound to constrain, to some degree, respondents' capacities to describe themselves in terms that capture their identities. Perhaps more significantly for the discussion at this point, identities are more dynamic and complex than conventional British conceptions of ethnic difference allow and there is evidence that significant processes are afoot which are increasingly challenging many taken for granted assumptions about ethnic, and for that matter national, identities. Nor are these processes confined to the identities of Britain's minority ethnic citizens.

Thus many commentators have noted how the process of devolution is leading to a reinvigoration of longstanding national identities among both the Scots and the Welsh. Hand in hand with devolution is a growing regional agenda, at both national and EU levels, which has the potential to reawaken regional identities, which have long appeared dormant. An interesting by-product of these developments has been the way in which Englishness as an identity has been increasingly problematised (McCrone, 2000). As the dominant national group in Britain, it was not necessary until recently for most English people to reflect upon the relationship between English and British identities. With the increasing assertiveness of other national identities within Britain, however, the English are being forced to confront the question of what exactly marks them off. This was reflected, in the later years of the twentieth century in a flurry of television programmes and press commentary on the question 'Who are the English?'.

Interestingly, this appears to be a novel question only if we lack an historical perspective. As Linda Colley has shown in her major study *Britons* (1992), the British nation was invented in the wake of the 1707 Act of Union. It was forged as a national identity in and through a series of conflicts, notably with France, over a period of about a century and a half. So successful was this process that, until brought into question by the recent developments, the existence of a British national identity was rarely, if ever, challenged. Yet it was quintessentially a political project in which a new set of essentially ethnic boundaries was consciously erected and celebrated.

The instrumental character of this process draws our attention to the fact that current attempts to rediscover some primordial essence of an *English* identity are fundamentally misplaced. As Colin Kidd has shown (1999) in the 17$^{th}$ Century there were at least eight versions of the English story - all of them related to different political projects ranging from Royalism to Leveller radicalism. A common problem for all of them was how to weave the diverse histories of the various groups out of which England had emerged, into a coherent national story. It was not an easy task. As late as 1867, *The Times* noted:

> ... there is hardly such a thing as a pure Englishman in this island. In place of the rather vulgarised and very inaccurate phrase, Anglo-Saxon, our national denomination, to be strictly correct, would be a composite of a dozen national titles ... (quoted in Walvin, 1984; 19).

But if the questions of what constitutes a British or English identity are not new, they are no less real for those who find it necessary to confront them at the beginning of the 21st century.

Of course, these discussions have characteristically been framed in terms of *nationality* rather than *ethnicity*. However, given what was said above about the construction of ethnic difference in Britain, this increasing problematisation of British identity is of great significance, since it undermines the dualistic majority/minority couple and, at least in principle, opens the way for a more sophisticated understanding of ethnic difference and diversity. On the other hand, however, it may lead to a defensiveness about identities thought to be under threat which could reinforce exclusionary pressures. The furious negative press reaction to the Parekh report on the *Future of Multi-Ethnic Britain* (2000) may be an example of this latter process at work.

This Janus-faced potential of current developments arises because, conceptually, ethnicity is a matter both of self-identity ('we' statements) and of categorisation ('they' statements). Identity and categorisation do not proceed independently of one another but are mutually constitutive. In most societies some groups and individuals have a greater capacity than others to define the terms under which categorisations are made. As a consequence, self-identification takes place in contexts where others' categorisations to some extent constrain the choices that can realistically be made. In other words, if others do not accept one's identity choices it may, in practice, be difficult, if not impossible, to act out the implications of those choices.

In the British context, these kinds of constraints may take the form of subtle social cues and messages that constrain behaviour or they may take much more concrete forms, as in the persistence of high levels of racial violence and the operation of immigration law (see the discussion in Mason 2000). Similarly occupational segregation or exclusion may also mean that, notwithstanding their formal entitlement to full citizenship rights, many members of Britain's minority ethnic communities experience a sense of exclusion from the identity 'British'. It is against this background that we have to understand the complex and fundamental changes currently affecting the identities of Britain's minority ethnic citizens. Of particular note is the increasingly common laying claim to hybrid identities, such as Black-British and Pakistani-British, which challenge still further what was until recently an apparently unproblematic national category, unsullied with considerations of ethnic difference (Modood, 1997c. See also Parekh, 2000).

Evidence from the fourth PSI survey shows that Britain's minority ethnic citizens call on a wide variety of cultural and other characteristics in defining their ethnic identities. Respondents were asked to rank in importance a range of characteristics in terms of which they might describe themselves to strangers. These included: nationality, skin colour, country of origin, age, job, education, height, colour of hair or eyes, level of income and father's job. In other words, they included a range of more or less visible personal characteristics and attributes only some of which are conventionally associated with ethnicity. In particular, characteristics often used in the measurement of social class, such as job and education, scored highly among all minority ethnic groups. In addition, religion was of great significance, especially among members of the Asian groups. Put another way, it is clear that in constructing their identities, the respondents in the PSI survey utilised a range of physical, positional and lifestyle characteristics in combinations which both varied between groups but which also exhibited considerable similarities (Modood, 1997c: 290-338).

Nevertheless, there is also evidence that these identifications were made in the context of a recognition that others categorise them in a way which constrains the choices they themselves can make. A number of persons of Asian descent who responded to the PSI survey indicated that they were inclined to think of themselves as 'black' in situations where they were in contact with white people. Among the reasons given was the belief that this was how they were defined by whites - in other words, they felt their choices were constrained (Modood, 1997c: 295-6).

Having said this, it would equally be a mistake to believe that identities are static or that Britain's minority ethnic citizens are simply passive victims in the face of economic exclusion and racist attitudes and behaviour. There are myriad examples ranging from self-help community organisations to various forms of political mobilisation of Britain's minority citizens challenging their exclusion. More subtly there is considerable evidence of a process of continuous change in the ways the identities of Britain's varied citizens are constructed and negotiated. Modood has attempted to capture how, for second and third generation members of minority ethnic groups in Britain, subtle and complex changes in patterns of ethnic identification have occurred. His analysis suggests that there is no straightforward relationship between 'the cultural content of an ethnicity and strategies of ethnic self-definition' (Modood, 1997c: 337). The result is a shift from what he calls 'behavioural difference' to an emphasis on 'associational identity':

> for many the strength of their ethnic identity was owed to a group pride in response to perceptions of racial exclusion and ethnic stereotyping by the white majority. The consequent sense of rejection and insecurity was instrumental in assertions of ethnic identities, often in forms susceptible to forging new anti-racist solidarities (such as 'black') and hyphenated (such as British-Pakistani) or even multiple identities (Modood, 1997c: 337).

Modood suggests that the resultant identifications are much less taken for granted than those of earlier generations (based on shared cultural values) and more consciously chosen, publicly celebrated and debated; part of a contested arena of identity politics. As a result, they are potentially fluid and more open to change with political and other circumstances, sometimes reviving old cultural practices, sometimes generating new ones (Modood, 1997c: 337).

What this suggests is that changing identities are intimately bound up with patterns of inclusion and exclusion. Patterns of upward occupational mobility, or those of labour market or spacial segregation and exclusion, create different opportunities and pressures. Individual and collective identity choices are made in the context of these complex patterns of opportunity and constraint. These in turn impact on educational and occupational aspirations, as Modood's analysis of what he calls the 'ethnic minorities' drive for qualifications' demonstrates (see the discussion above and Modood, 1998). It is against this background that we have to understand the context within which health service recruitment takes place and the dilemmas facing those who would wish to push forward the equality agenda in the NHS.

## Differential Recruitment in the Nursing Workforce: Exclusion or Choice?

As we have seen, in the nurse education centres studied in the research, there was a tendency to regard disproportionately low levels of application from some minority ethnic groups, and the consequentially small numbers of nurses drawn from Asian minority ethnic groups, as being essentially a matter of choice. That is, it was widely assumed that applicants failed to materialise from these groups mainly because of processes operating within the groups themselves. Among the explanations invoked were a lack of understanding of the opportunities available or of the nature of nursing; parental pressure; language and qualification deficits; and presumed cultural prohibitions or preferences. It was this attribution of responsibility to the groups themselves that in part explained the relative paucity of initiatives to target members of these groups and the uncertainties expressed by respondents about how best such targeting might be pursued. As a result, our research was able to identify few effective initiatives to address the marked under-representation of Asian minority ethnic groups in the nursing workforce that our research revealed.

We are conscious that statistical representativeness, measured in the manner suggested in our research, is not the only way in which to conceptualise equality. There is a large literature which draws attention to the different ways in which equal opportunities may be conceived and, hence, to the different potential measures of their successful achievement (Jewson and Mason, 1986; Cockburn, 1989; Jewson and Mason, 1994; Bagilhole, 1997. See also the discussion in Chapter 8). Moreover, even where members of different groups are represented in proportion to their presence in the population, it may still be the case that other qualified candidates are denied access on the basis of discriminatory practices. Indeed, this is one of the arguments often levelled against the use of quotas. The representativeness conception of equality also ignores the possibility that some of the differences between groups may result from differential occupational aspirations and choices (Edwards, 1995: 9-10). Having entered these caveats, however, it is important to remember that the key point at issue in our research was the contrast between nationally articulated aspirations and local understandings and practices. In point of fact, the institutions we studied could have felt confident in defending a mismatch between their profile and that of the population as a whole only if they could be certain it were not to be explained by a failure to have effective equal opportunities provisions. As we have seen, in most cases they had not even the means to know whether such a mismatch existed.

On the other hand we also noted above that there was evidence of significant levels of upward occupational and social mobility among Britain's minority ethnic communities. We also adduced evidence that revealed high levels of post-16 educational participation and of aspiration – what Modood calls a 'drive for qualification'. Against this background, it is at least possible that well-qualified minority ethnic citizens do not aspire to a nursing career because they have set their sights higher – either in terms of occupational status or, perhaps crucially, income. This issue is not, of course, an easy one to unravel. Choice and constraint are not, after all, entirely independent of one another. There is also little reason to believe that people aspire to occupations from which they expect, by one means or another, to be excluded. There is little reason to be confident that existing equal opportunities provisions have effectively eliminated discriminatory selection decision-making from the nursing profession, or from the health service more generally. As a result we have no way of knowing whether occupational choices would be exercised differently in a more meritocratic environment. Moreover, the evidence adduced above in Chapter 2 about the persistence of racist practices in the NHS might suggest that those able to do so might avoid choosing occupations likely to expose them to such experiences.

The question remains, however, of what the consequences for policy development might be if under-representation were, indeed, to turn out to be a consequence of differential occupational choices among different ethnic groups and that such choices persisted even in the absence of racism and discrimination. This is a question that is not confined to the nursing and midwifery professions. Similar issues also confront a number of other occupations where the under-representation of minority ethnic groups persists.

Dandeker and Mason (2001) have recently considered some of these issues in the context of the armed services where there is also a mismatch between the personnel profile and that of the population as a whole. Here they note that equal opportunities commitments are characteristically expressed differently in the case of minority ethnic groups and women. In the case of the former, there is an explicit commitment to transforming the personnel profile so that it reflects the ethnic profile of the population as a whole. In the case of women, by contrast, the commitment is to greater equality of opportunity to serve with no expectation that the numbers of women serving in the armed services will ever be proportional to those in the population as a whole. Dandeker and Mason suggest that this contrast implicitly invokes two different senses of 'representativeness': the statistical and the delegative. In the latter, members of groups are represented in the ranks of any profession by some of their members but this does not require proportional representation. Given that delegative representation for women appears to be widely accepted in the context of the armed services,[5] they ask whether this might not also be the way forward in the event that differential occupational choices made it impossible to meet existing targets for minority ethnic recruitment. Dandeker and Mason acknowledge that such a solution would be vulnerable to charges of tokenism. However, they note that the currently fashionable concept of diversity, in at least some of its dominant guises, does provide a legitimation for such a strategy. In the context of the armed services, they suggest that the embracing of diversity is hindered by a number of cultural and organisational barriers. They suggest that these have their roots not only in the traditions of the armed services themselves but also in key aspects of the British national myth, and its associated conceptions of national belonging and ethnic difference; issues which we touched upon above.

There is not space here, nor is it appropriate, to pursue this discussion of the armed services further. It is appropriate to note, however, that the concept of diversity is widely promoted in some equal opportunities circles as a solution to some persistent dilemmas and as a way of overcoming organisational resistance to policy implementation. In the final chapter, we revisit some of the key arguments for greater equity, consider some of the dilemmas to which they give rise and explore their implications for the pursuit of greater equity in the NHS.

## Notes

1 The 2001 Census contained a revised question that did offer respondents selecting 'White' a further sub-set of choices. This might be seen as a recognition of the problematic character of the category, and its uncertain relationship to people's identities. However, it is equally arguable that the change was driven in the first instance as much by an effective campaign for recognition by some sections of the Irish-descended community in London as by any significant rethinking of the category. The new categories did, however, permit greater opportunities for recording mixed origins and for affirming 'hybrid' identities. Having said this, there is to date, little evidence that these revisions have been reflected in a more sophisticated understanding of ethnic diversity in most policy making circles.

2 Scares about immigration and the presence of aliens are not, of course, a purely post Second World War phenomenon (Mason, 2000: 24).

3 The irony that they, too, have been forced to work with the same categories is not lost on the authors. Indeed, this illustrates the difficulties facing any researcher or policy maker working in this area. Some of the implications of this situation are considered in more detail in Chapter 8. In the meantime, we would defend our earlier analysis of admissions and selection practices by noting that the key point at issue in that discussion was the mismatch between national policy commitments and the pattern of day to day practice on the ground. As we have argued, this mismatch, was a result both of structural factors and failures of political will. Nevertheless, we believe that the kinds of questions we are raising in this chapter do have significant implications for attempts to find a way to transcend the limitations of current policy.

4 This is not least because data from the fourth PSI study (Modood *et al.*, 1997) show that occupational mobility does not feed through in any straightforward way to enhanced life chances. Data on household incomes, for example, show that only Chinese households had incomes close to those of whites while Caribbean, Indian and African Asian household were all more likely than whites to experience poverty and were less likely to have large family incomes. These results lead to an important qualification to the evidence on upward occupational mobility. When household incomes are taken into account, African Asians and Indians fare less well than those of Chinese descent, while Caribbeans are much better placed than Pakistanis and Bangladeshis (Berthoud 1997: 180). These data thus provide further reasons to be cautious in assessing the significance of occupational mobility and the relative labour market placement of groups.

5 They point out that not even in the feminist literature is proportionality seen as an appropriate goal.

# 8 Policy, Politics and Health Care

We concluded chapter 7 by questioning what would be the policy consequences of a discovery that the under-representation of some minority ethnic groups in the nursing and midwifery workforce turned out to be a consequence of conscious occupational choice-making on the part of those involved. Whatever caveats we enter about the relationship between choice and constraint, and however much we acknowledge the power of exclusionary processes and negative experiences, this must remain at least a theoretical possibility. To presume otherwise is, in fact, to fall victim to a new variant of the assimilationist assumptions which have long permeated health policy in the U.K. Given that the association of equity with proportional representation is close to being an orthodoxy in many equal opportunities circles, this may seem a dramatic claim. In point of fact, however, it is merely to highlight one of a number of persistent dilemmas in the history of equal opportunities theory and practice.

## Recurrent Dilemmas of Equal Opportunities

Debates about equal opportunities, and more generally those about the nature of equality, have a long history, embracing a range of complex philosophical, political and moral issues, to which it is not possible to do justice here (see, for example, Edwards, 1995). There are, however, two recurrent dilemmas which have regularly dogged not just intellectual debate but also day to day policy development and which have particular relevance for this discussion.

The first is the question of whether the objective of policy should be to secure equality of *opportunity* or equality of *outcome*. The dominant emphasis in Britain has been on equality of opportunity with the proceduralist focus characteristic of what has become known as the 'liberal' model of equal opportunities (Jewson and Mason, 1986; Jewson *et al.*, 1995; Jewson and Mason, 1994). Here it is argued that equality can be achieved if the skills and qualities of individuals, which are assumed to be randomly distributed in the population, can be matched more precisely to the functional requirements of occupational roles. The emphasis, then, is on the bureaucratic regulation of recruitment and selection systems designed to remove unfair, and inefficient, barriers to the achievement of that aim (Jewson and Mason, 1986; Mason, 1990b). The individualist emphasis of the liberal model also means that equality of opportunity is characteristically structured in terms of the opportunity for people, whether men or women and of whatever ethnicity, to be treated *as if they were the same*. No explicit account is taken of the possibility that there may be systematic differences between people which have their origins in group membership.

The limitations of this model are well known and do not require detailed rehearsal here. We may note in particular, however, that this approach takes no account of the way in which extra-labour market issues intrude into the process of matching individual attributes to the functional requirements of roles as, for example, when domestic obligations lead to discontinuous careers for women (Rees, 1992). More fundamentally, the very conceptions of skill on which the liberal model is based take no account of the way in which definitions of skill are gendered (Webb and Liff, 1988).

In practice, as Jewson and Mason (1986) have pointed out, such proceduralist policies have frequently been judged in terms of standards that are, in principle, the province of an outcomes-centred approach – what Jewson and Mason call the radical model. In its extreme form such a perspective would entail positive discrimination in favour of under-represented groups, a practice which is unlawful in Britain. However, as we have seen, much orthodox equal opportunities discourse entails making comparisons between groups in terms of the notion of proportionality of representation. Hence the stress on monitoring, measurement and intervention in terms of positive action even if, as we have argued, research evidence suggests that these have by no means been widespread even among organisations apparently committed to equal opportunities (Jewson *et al.*, 1992; 1995; Iganski, *et al.*, 1998). We are faced, then, with a paradox that the liberal model's emphasis on opportunity is frequently combined with a concern with outcomes while, in practice, the measures necessary to deliver greater equity in outcomes are not systematically pursued. This was precisely the situation revealed by the research reported in Chapter 6. Jewson and Mason (1986) suggest that one source of this paradox is the frequent failure thoroughly to think through the implications of juxtaposing contrasting principles of equity and criteria of success. As we shall see below, however, it is also possible that a further set of conceptual weaknesses concerning the arguments characteristically employed to promote equal opportunities is also implicated.

Before we proceed to a discussion of these matters, however, it is necessary briefly to review the second recurrent and related dilemma. This is the question of whether equal opportunities can be addressed through the medium of generic policies or whether advancing the cause of equity requires different policies and practices in respect of the inequalities experienced by different disadvantaged groups (such as women, minority ethnic groups or those with disabilities).

There is widespread recognition that the precise nature of the disadvantage experienced by different marginalised and excluded groups varies in both character and degree. This fact is characteristically stressed forcefully by political activists. Nevertheless, with limited exceptions, equal opportunities policies in both the private and public sectors have tended to take a generic form. Where differences in the needs of particular groups have been recognised this has tended to be reflected in targeted positive action provisions (Jewson *et al.*, 1990; 1992; 1995). This contrast is mirrored at government policy level. Despite significant differences in the legislative provisions regarding sex, race and, more recently, disability discrimination (Bourne and Whitmore, 1996), official Employment Department (now Department for Education and Employment) advice on the development of equal opportunities policies has generally focused on generic recommendations (U.K. Employment Department, 1991).

There are often practical reasons for the adoption of generic policies (Jewson *et al.*, 1995). These include pressure on resources that are characteristically limited and often contested within organisations. In addition there are often variations in the perceived legitimacy of the claims of different groups. This may give rise to the argument that generic policies offer the opportunity to piggy-back the needs of less favoured groups on the acceptance of general principles justified by reference to the better recognised or accepted needs of others. Over and above these practical considerations, however, the choice of generic policy is often dictated by the more or less explicit embracing by policy makers of the liberal conception of equal opportunities.

By contrast, the insistent political demands of women, minority ethnic groups and, more recently, those with disabilities are more likely to stress the distinctive needs and problems of these groups. Such demands are counterposed to the ultimately liberal, individualist focus of generic policies and have helped to ensure the survival of a group-centred equality agenda. This in turn has led to demands for more effective monitoring and measurement, and has bolstered arguments for targeting and other forms of positive action. Critically, these features highlight the weaknesses of approaches to equal opportunities that concentrate on technical or administrative solutions and they signal the ultimately political character of equal opportunities as an issue for excluded and marginalised groups. We return to this question of the political status of equal opportunities below.

Despite the dominance of generic approaches to policy, however, it is by no means the case that, in practice, such policies have pursued the needs of all groups with equal vigour. Jewson *et al.* (1992; 1995), for example, identify a number of cases where equal opportunities for women have been, in practice, higher up the agenda than the needs of minority ethnic groups. Moreover, in the case of the armed services discussed in Chapter 7, it is clear that explicitly different policy agendas have been embraced in respect of gender and race equality (Dandeker and Mason, 2001). Even where such explicit contrasts are not spelt out, however, differences of emphasis are not difficult to discern – most notably in what is frequently not said. In this connection, it is interesting to note that the question of gender equality in the nursing profession is rarely, if ever, constructed in terms of the problem of achieving a proportional representation of men. Instead, the focus is more usually on the disproportionate numbers of men in senior positions, relative to their presence in the profession as a whole. Once again, the contrast with the way equity for minority ethnic groups is conceived is palpable, emphasising yet again some difficult questions about how we conceptualise occupational choice and constraint. As in the military example, this raises the question of the utility of the concept of diversity which, as we shall see, has been gaining ground in equal opportunities circles as a potential solution to some of the persistent dilemmas outlined above.

## Fragmenting Identities and the Concept of Diversity

In Chapter 7 we noted that there was evidence of an increasing volatility in the opportunities and identity choices open to members of all ethnic groups. These developments have proceeded hand in hand with developments in intellectual and political discourse. Thus, in the last 10 to 15 years, the conceptions of groups and categories – and the presumptions of shared interest that underlie them – which have been central to much equal opportunities thought have come under sustained pressure. Perhaps the earliest manifestation came from feminists who, from the early 1980s onwards, attacked essentialised conceptions of woman (see, for example, the vigorous debate in the pages of *Feminist Review* from 1984 onwards). Some of the most trenchant challenges came from black feminists who attacked what they saw as the dominance of white middle class perspectives. They argued that patriarchal oppression was mediated by racism, making the experience and opportunities of black and white women quite different (see, for example, Amos and Parmar, 1984; Ware, 1991). At the same time, other writers in the feminist tradition have challenged the essentialisation of *ethnic* difference, arguing that ethnicity is gendered in ways which both differentiate the experience of men and women but which are also constitutive of ethnic differences themselves (Anthias and Yuval-Davis, 1992: 113-115. See also Afshah and Maynard, 1994; Bradley, 1996: 107-112; Brah, 1996). A further challenge came from Tariq Modood who, in a celebrated article, challenged the use of the political category 'black' as a generic label for all who were seen as victims of white exclusionary practices. Such a practice, he argued, failed to capture the specificity of either Asian experiences or identities and, in so doing, substituted an illusion of political unity for a genuine attempt to address the realities of diverse day to day experiences of racism (Modood, 1988; 1992. See also the discussion in Mason, 1990a; 1992).

In some ways more fundamental challenges to conventional conceptions of groups and categories have come from developments in social theory associated with postmodernist and post-structuralist thought. According to this view, the pace of change in the (post)modern world, together with an ever-expanding array of choices and possibilities, creates conditions in which individuals are increasingly freed to make multiple identity choices which match the purposes (or even the whims) of the moment. In other words, old-style, modernist explanations of the social world in terms of large-scale and relatively stable social categories do violence to the complexity of the everyday experiences of individuals in the post-modern world. (For a useful discussion of these issues, see Bradley, 1996: 21-27. See also Rattansi and Westwood, 1994.) By emphasising difference, diversity and identity, such theorisations make it much easier to recognise the conditional and situational character of people's identities. They also allow us to take cognisance of the ways in which ethnicity, gender, class and age (to name but a few key aspects of identity) may interact in complex and changing ways to structure people's images of themselves and others. Examples of this process at work were revealed in the findings of the fourth PSI study discussed in Chapter 7.

Postmodernism, then, identifies, in the diverse identity options open to individuals, the opportunity to challenge the stereotyping and categorisation all too often characteristic of the behaviour of 'ethnic majorities' (see the discussion in Jenkins, 1997: 29-30). At the same time it challenges the essentialisation of the ethnic, gender and other categories that have been central to the process of constructing, but also of measuring and tracking, conventionally defined social inequalities.

These challenges to the conceptions of groups and categories conventionally underpinning the equal opportunities agenda have coincided with the emergence of the concept of diversity in management thought and rhetoric. (See, for example, Herriot and Pemberton, 1995; Jackson and Associates, 1992; Kandola and Fullerton, 1998; Kandola, Fullerton, and Ahmed, 1995; Kossek and Lobel, 1996; Liff 1996; Thomas, 1991; Wheatley and Griffiths, 1997.) The concept came to Britain from the United States where it had become extensively popularised in the equal employment opportunities literature in the late 1980s and early 1990s (notably in an influential book by Thomas [1991]). It seems first to have appeared in a U.K. context in organisations which had either United States parent companies or extensive U.S. operations (see, for example, the discussion of Mineralco in Jewson *et al.*, 1995).

Diversity, it is claimed, entails a radical reconceptualisation of the equal opportunities agenda. In this model people are valued because of their differences. It is committed to using fully the talents of all members of the workforce, allowing them to rise to the limit of their abilities. The diversity model is thus said simultaneously to address the needs of every individual in the workforce and to deliver operational benefits to the organisation as a whole. Because it no longer focuses exclusively on those groups deemed in some way to be disadvantaged or under-represented, it offers advantages to all employees, including white men, and thus engages their commitment rather than promoting their resentment (Kandola and Fullerton, 1998; Kandola, Fullerton, and Ahmed, 1995; Thomas, 1991). Diversity, then, is said to represent the central organising concept in the emergence of a new receptiveness to equal opportunities within the business community.

Whether such optimistic prognoses can be realised depends, of course, on the degree to which commitment to the diversity paradigm is real rather than merely rhetorical (a new name for old actions or inactions). Like old-style equal opportunities policies, it also depends on the effectiveness of the organisational arrangements for delivering on policy commitments. More fundamentally, it depends on the outcome of some unresolved uncertainties about the precise meaning and implications of diversity. (For a rather different analysis of the range of approaches embraced by the term see Liff, 1996.)

The concept of diversity, as it is typically encountered in organisational settings in both Britain and the United States, has two distinct resonances. On the one hand it has a specifically *individual* focus. In this conceptualisation (which is the dominant one in Britain) modern business operates most effectively when it harnesses the diverse talents of all the *individuals* who make up the team. This involves not merely drawing on a diverse range of technical skills. It also entails valuing and harnessing the distinctive personal characteristics and thinking which different individuals may bring to the table, generating new and creative solutions to problems from clashes of views and styles.

On the other hand, the term diversity may also have a distinctly collective resonance. Thus it is often argued that women, *as women*, bring distinctive values, skills of interaction and ways of thinking to the team. Similarly, it is sometimes claimed that people from diverse cultural backgrounds can also contribute new and valued inputs to the process of team deliberation by bringing personal characteristics, ways of thinking and modes of interaction that are *collective* in origin. In other words, then, what is being argued is that characteristics that were once seen as problematic because they embodied *difference* from the 'normal' and familiar, are now to be valued for the same reason.

There is little doubt that the individualist version of diversity is the dominant one in Britain (see, Kandola, Fullerton, and Ahmed, 1995: 31). In this guise, equal opportunities policy focuses on the empowerment of individuals rather than being directed to the problems of specific minorities. It is a conceptualisation that leaves little room for the recognition of the collective sources of disadvantage which have been of concern to the conventional equal opportunities agenda. This relative dominance of the individualist version of diversity in Britain reflects the different historical, demographic and political situations of the U.S. and the U.K. (Mason, 1990b: 84-5). In the USA the collective resonance of diversity is more strongly underpinned by political and demographic realities, arguments associated with marketing and by the group-centredness of U.S. coalition politics.[1] Its emergence was underpinned by a well-established climate of federal contract compliance requirements and relatively robust anti-discrimination legislation. It was, however, given a further boost by the publication of *Workforce 2000* (U.S. Department of Labor, 1987) which predicted that white males would constitute a minority of those entering the labour force by the beginning of the new century (Jackson and Associates, 1992). To these labour supply concerns were added a recognition that the U.S. domestic market was becoming equally diverse while the pace of globalisation was apparently quickening. A diverse workforce thus had marketing advantages by incorporating a range of skills and cultural sensitivities which allowed the organisation more accurately to identify changing patterns of demand while presenting itself as attuned to diverse customer needs (Thomas, 1991: 3-7). The key to progress in the United States then, however halting and conditional, has been power – political and economic.[2] Whether the same conditions apply in the United Kingdom is less certain. In the remainder of the chapter we explore the implications of the foregoing discussion for our theme of equal opportunities in the National Health Service.

## Evaluating Arguments for Equal Opportunities in the NHS

As we have seen, two broad kinds of arguments are commonly used to support equal opportunity measures in the field of employment. They are, respectively, those that appeal to considerations of equity and fairness, and those that rely upon appeals to self-interest or pragmatism (often referred to as a 'business case'). The two kinds of arguments are often used in tandem. For example, in 1993, the Secretary of State for Health argued, in the Foreword to the Programme of Action on Ethnic Minority Staff in the National Health Service, that: '... taking action to promote equality in employment is not just a matter of moral fairness to people from minority ethnic groups. It is good, sound common sense, and it makes good business sense too' (U.K. Department of Health 1993).

The use of pragmatic, or utilitarian, arguments for policy implementation has been a central characteristic of the 'political economy' of equal opportunities in Britain in the 1980s and 1990s (see Jewson and Mason 1994). The alleged business, rather than moral, benefits of policy have been promoted, in large part because of a belief that managerial practices are more likely to be shaped by enlightened self-interest than a concern for social justice.

Against this background it is noteworthy that the various available arguments and rationales for enhanced equal opportunities provision were neither fully and widely understood nor wholeheartedly embraced in the institutions studied in our research. This is partly a matter of the effectiveness with which the message of national policy commitments and their rationale had been disseminated. It relates directly to arrangements for communication, education and training - particularly of those staff involved in recruitment and selection. It may, however, also point to limitations in both of the kinds of argument, identified above, in terms of which equal opportunities measures are characteristically justified.

With regard to arguments based on morality and justice, all the centres studied espoused a formal commitment to equality of opportunity. Yet it is clear from the interview data that, even if they were wholeheartedly committed to this principle (and we have no way of judging whether this was the case) not all respondents drew the same lessons for policy development. The persistent confusion encountered among many respondents between positive action and positive discrimination may be interpreted as a matter of ignorance and lack of understanding. Yet it may equally reflect a genuine difference of view about the nature of equality, and the measures by which it may legitimately be pursued which, as we saw above, has a long intellectual history. In other words, the limitation of the moral argument for equality of opportunity and positive action is that it embodies principles which have contradictory resonances and implications, even for those predisposed to respond to morally based arguments (Jewson and Mason 1986; Cockburn 1989; Jewson and Mason 1994; Lloyd 1994; Edwards 1995; Bagilhole 1997).

This difficulty is one reason, of course, why much of the policy literature emphasises instead the pragmatic or business case for equal opportunities. It also underpins some of the arguments about the advantages of the diversity paradigm. Linked to this is the argument that busy managers, with a variety of operational objectives to meet, are more likely to be persuaded by arguments which emphasise the practical benefits, to their business objectives, of the measures proposed. Additionally, it is sometimes argued that they are also more receptive to arguments framed in terms of the rhetoric of their everyday working lives (Jewson and Mason, 1991). The limitation of these kinds of argument for equal opportunities and positive action is that they can, all too easily, lead to the opposite conclusion from that anticipated by those who promote them. Indeed, Michael Rubenstein has argued provocatively that if there were, indeed, a convincing business case for equal opportunities, managers would already have embraced it. That it still needs to be promoted is, for him, evidence of its basic weakness (Rubenstein 1987).[3] Whether this is the case or not, it is clear that, in our case studies, some recruiters were pursuing those sources of applicants which they expected to permit them to reach their targets, without regard to some of the wider labour supply arguments adduced in support of targeting minority ethnic communities. To the extent that they were able to successfully recruit the required numbers without such targeting, we should perhaps not be surprised if they were less than fully convinced by the need to take other steps. In addition, we should note that managers have a number of different targets and objectives to meet. Again we should not be surprised if the operational objectives of meeting recruitment targets, delivering nurse education to an appropriate standard and, more generally, assuring effective patient care take precedence in their priority setting over activities which, from this perspective, are more long-term or peripheral. (Compare the case study of 'Retailco' in Jewson *et al.* 1995.)

What this suggests is that the business case for equal opportunities and positive action requires to be underpinned and bolstered by moral arguments for social justice if it is not to swept away by changes in circumstances.[4] Moreover, given the scope for individual variations in interpretations of both the business and moral cases, it is clear that individual commitment and initiative cannot be relied upon to deliver long-term systematic change. As has long been recognised (see for example, Jewson *et al.* 1990), such change requires commitment from those in organisations with the power to enforce policy change, monitor performance and deploy rewards and sanctions. In the case of the NHS this implies more than simply rhetorical commitment on the part of government. As the case of nurse recruitment demonstrates only too clearly, the problem for such an effective policy thrust in the NHS is its fragmented organisational structure. Nurses, as we have seen, are trained under programmes accredited by the ENB. They are educated by nurse education centres that are typically departments, or faculties, of self-governing universities. Applicants may apply for training places through the ENB or direct to centres. Once trained, they are subsequently employed by self-governing NHS Trusts which contract with education centres for the provision of training places. Trusts, in turn, have a variety of operational and financial concerns which will affect the degree to which they assign high priority to equal opportunities matters. In these circumstances, the translation of national level commitments into effective local policy would appear to require a pattern of central target setting and monitoring, and a range of potential sanctions, which there is as yet little evidence to suggest is high on the agenda.

In addition, we would suggest, it also means developing a more convincing method of linking the business and moral cases for equal opportunities than those that focus simply on questions of recruitment and retention. One possibility is that a focus on effective service delivery might provide a vehicle for establishing such a connection by espousing the potential benefits of an ethnically diverse workforce.

A link between the recruitment of health service workers from minority ethnic communities and the provision of services sensitive to the needs of those communities has long been recognised in health policy circles and has been emphasised in a number of influential studies and policy documents. Thus the King's Fund Equal Opportunities Task Force, established by the Department of Health in the late 1980s to develop equal opportunities expertise for health services, argued that: 'We believe that by ensuring equal opportunities in employment for ethnic minorities, Authorities will be better placed to improve the delivery of service to minority racial groups' (1987: 3). The National Association of Health Authorities also argued, in its report *Action Not Words* (1988), that: 'An effective way of making health services responsive to the needs of a multi-racial and multi-cultural population is to ensure that members of minority ethnic groups are employed at all levels in the health service and thus involved automatically in the planning, management and delivery of those services' (1988: 10). More recently, the overall aim of the programme of action on ethnic minority staff in the NHS - launched in December 1993 - is to achieve 'the equitable representation of minority ethnic groups at all levels in the NHS ... reflecting the ethnic composition of the local population', on the principle that: 'Failure to do so could result in a "eurocentric" model of health care which does not deliver a satisfactory level of service to patients from minority ethnic groups' (U.K. Dept. of Health 1993: 4, and Foreword). The arguments for workforce diversity have also been echoed beyond the provision of health care in the areas of policing (Etzioni, 1997), business (Pandaya, 1997; Ross and Schneider, 1992), criminal justice (Rose, 1997), and the military (Joyce, 1997).

## Equal Opportunities in Employment and Service Delivery: Compatible Objectives?

Having made this point, however, we should note that simply to assert the mutual benefits to be derived from the pursuit of equality in the fields both of employment and service delivery does not, of itself, ensure that either is effectively delivered. This is because a key question is the precise mechanism by which greater workforce diversity leads to better service delivery to a diverse patient pool.

There is a substantial literature that draws attention to deficiencies in the care offered to minority ethnic groups in the modern NHS. (See, for example, Bowler, 1993; Gerrish *et al.*, 1996; Johnson, 1993; Mason 2000.

For a wider perspective see Leininger, 1991.) Not all of those identifying the problem, however, offer the same solution. Implicit in the policy pronouncements reviewed in the previous section is the assumption that minority ethnic staff are better placed to respond to the health care needs of minority ethnic patients. There are a range of reasons why this might be the case. Thus, it might be said that minority ethnic staff are better placed to communicate with co-ethnics, either in terms of specific language skills or because of their appreciation of the cultural subtexts of particular linguistic formulations. Additionally, it may be argued that they are more alert to culturally specific non-verbal cues or culturally approved modes of emotional display. It is arguable that such processes in part underlie some of the systematic failures of understanding revealed in Bowler's (1993) study of maternity care. Alternatively such staff might be expected to be more alive to particular cultural requirements, preferences and prohibitions. As a result, they may be perceived to be more acceptable to minority ethnic patients as carers, at least in certain intimate or culturally significant contexts.

All of these scenarios are highly plausible and it would not be difficult to identify examples of how each might operate in practice. The implication would appear to be that the ideal care scenario is one that offered the potential for ethnic matching of carers and patients. However, it is equally easy to identify a number of potential problems with this approach. An obvious operational problem is that of ensuring that the ethnically 'appropriate' staff were always available, at the time needed, by each patient. This would be difficult to guarantee even if there were a complete match between the patient and staff profile of each hospital and other treatment unit. More significantly from the point of view of the argument in Chapter 7, it presumes that there are mechanisms by which we could measure ethnic difference in a sufficiently fine tuned manner to achieve such a situation, even were a wide range of recruits to come forward. This problem is made more complex still by two other features to which we have already drawn attention. One is the apparently increasing volatility of ethnic identities. The second is the way in which ethnicity intersects with other dimensions of identity. In other words, patients seeking an exact match might be expected, in some circumstances, to be as exercised about the gender, class, status or other personal characteristics of carers as about their location in terms of conventional ethnic monitoring categories. Another way to put this is to remind ourselves, as the discussion in Chapter 7 and also above should have made plain, that identities are complex, socially achieved constructions. Even when ethnicity is salient, therefore, it is not the only determinant of our behaviour or our reactions to others (see the discussion in Gerrish *et al.*, 1996: 18-20 and in Mason, 2000: 11-14). All of this suggests that ethnic matching in any strict sense is a practical and conceptual impossibility.

This issue also raises the question of whether the service delivery (conceived in this way) and the employment agendas are entirely compatible. In fact it is arguable that, in each case, there are different pressures at work. In the context of the discussion in Chapter 7 about differential occupational choice-making, we should reflect on the possibility that pursuing the proportional representation agenda could, in practice, amount to an attempt to persuade people to do jobs that they would prefer to avoid. If this seems a rather dramatic way to pose the problem, we should at least recognise that there is evidence that minority ethnic staff can, all to easily, find themselves marginalised into particular roles. Gerrish *et al.* write of the danger of them being seen as 'a means of solving particular difficulties encountered in caring for minority ethnic clients, the most notable of these being the difficulties of communication', and often reduced to the roles of interpreters (1996: 142).

Given the difficulties that are posed by any suggestion of ethnic matching, the most obvious alternative approach to rendering culturally sensitive care is that which entails the educational preparation of nurses and other health service staff for working with an ethnically diverse patient population. Evidence from the study by Gerrish *et al.* (1996) suggests that, despite pockets of good practice and commitment, relatively slow progress has been made in Britain in adapting the nurse education curriculum to meet the challenges of nursing in a multi-ethnic society. Clearly, there is much that could be done, both to promote more sophisticated knowledge of other cultures, and to encourage a more flexible and reflexive approach on the part of practitioners. In particular, it may well be that there are generic communicative skills that can be deployed, maximising the adaptability of carers in problem solving in cross-cultural interactions (Gerrish *et al.*, 1996: 26-30. See also Leininger, 1991). Alongside these are those competencies that arise from a specific understanding of the requirements of others' cultures. Clearly, much could be done to prepare professionals for practice in an ethnically diverse environment by imparting appropriate knowledge and by developing the skills necessary to acquire new understandings while in practice (Gerrish *et al.*, 1996: 26-30. See also Leininger, 1991). Nevertheless, as we have seen, the NHS operates in an increasingly diverse environment, in which the parameters of ethnic identity, and their associated cultural practices, are themselves constantly shifting (Modood, 1997c: 337). As a consequence, the possibility of any individual carer encountering a situation for which she or he is unprepared must remain high, with all the potential this has to severely disrupt the interaction and adversely affect care (Gerrish *et al.*, 1996: 26).

Once again, then, we may doubt whether the solution to the problem can be allowed to rest entirely at an individual level; with the relationship between individual patient and carer. This is both because of the necessary limits to the range of appropriate knowledge any given nurse, or other professional, is likely to have and because, in any case, individual interactions are always mediated by other inter-personal processes. This suggests that a more appropriate focus may well be on the team. A diverse team will, by definition, always be able to deploy a wider range of knowledge, skills and competencies than any individual. This is widely recognised in the health service in terms of technical competencies and specialisms. There is no reason, in principle, why it should not be extended to the communicative and other inter-personal competencies that are the *sine qua non* of effective health care delivery. This suggests that the concept of diversity which we have touched on in several places above may, indeed, provide a way of thinking about the relationship between health service employment and service delivery that could address some of the dilemmas and difficulties considered in this chapter.

Diverse teams may, then, provide the mechanism to maximise culturally sensitive care and optimally meet the diverse needs of patients in Britain's multi-ethnic society. At the same time, the emphasis on diversity rather than proportionality of representation may provide a way of reconciling differential occupational choice with the equality agenda in employment. If it is to do so, however, two conditions must be met. The first is that the delegative representativeness that it embodies must not be allowed to lapse into a form of tokenism. Only if attempts continue to be made to ensure that differential recruitment is not a consequence of exclusionary processes in recruitment and selection will it be possible to be confident that genuine occupational choices are being exercised. The second is that the marginalisation of minority ethnic staff within diverse teams must be avoided. Their presence must not become an excuse for the failure of others to seek to acquire appropriate competencies and knowledge. Only then will the business advantages to the health service in service delivery terms be congruent with an equality agenda in the field of health service employment.

## Conclusion

We have argued elsewhere (Iganski *et al.*, 2001) that the character of the NHS as a key national institution, to which all political parties have recently reaffirmed commitment, may offer reason to be optimistic about the future of such an agenda. Its underlying principle of the provision of equitable and effective health care for all citizens provides a unique opportunity for the marriage of the moral and business cases, and hence for their mutual reinforcement. As we have seen, a key argument in support of enhanced diversity in the NHS workforce is the opportunity this offers to provide care more sensitive to the needs of patients from a variety of ethnic groups, and cultural and religious backgrounds. Providing sensitively and effectively for the health care needs of all Britain's citizens is integral to the mission of the NHS – it is a moral imperative rooted in a particular conception of social citizenship. It is now well recognised that delivery of this objective requires the embedding of a range of new competencies relevant to the needs of a diverse patient population. Attempts to change the ethnic profile of the NHS workforce in general and nurses in particular are widely seen as integral to this objective, however difficult they may prove to realise. At the very least, changes are required that ensure that minority ethnic recruits are not excluded or discouraged by the processes of recruitment and selection. The implications of this are that the moral imperatives of service delivery dictate the business case for equality of opportunity in NHS employment. If this rationale is accepted, what is required is an effective *national* strategy to overcome the difficulties posed by the current organisational fragmentation of the NHS.[5]

A key aspect of such a strategy would be a recognition that the diversity paradigm is not a magic solution to existing problems anymore than old style group-centred outcomes approaches that ignore differential choice and changing identities. It does not absolve policy makers from making difficult and ultimately political decisions. These might include accepting and working with differential occupational choice or accepting that, in some circumstances, the service delivery and employment equality agendas might come into conflict at least in the short term. A key initiative might well be a systematic raising of the status of the nursing profession, with the necessary remuneration consequences that this would have, to make it more attractive to those who currently eschew it as a career option.

More critically still, the NHS can realise its potential to advance the equality agenda only in the context of wider national progress in building a genuinely inclusive multi-ethnic society (see Dandeker and Mason, 2001) and by embracing the advantages of diversity in all aspects of national life (Mason, 2000).

## Notes

1 We should, however, note that even the group-centred version of diversity can be disadvantaging in so far as it may provide the context for the reproduction of stereotypes, such as those associated with women's domesticity or the exoticness of non-European cultures.

2 We are aware of the growth of challenges to traditional programmes of affirmative action in the United States. However, interviews with U.S. corporate personnel have indicated that the perceived business advantages of the continued pursuit of diversity is likely to maintain their commitment even were such challenges to reach an intensity and degree of success that has yet to be witnessed. (For a discussion of the debate around affirmative action, see Bowen and Bok, 1998.)

3 One objection to Rubenstein's argument, of course, is that managers are not necessarily rational. Consider the failings of British employers in the field of training in this regard. Unfortunately, however, this may not help us very much since, if managers are not rational, why should they be convinced by a case allegedly based on the pursuit of rational self-interest?

4 It is instructive to remember the fate of the 'demographic timebomb' - an anticipated downturn in labour supply resulting from earlier birthrate fluctuations - at the end of the 1980s. Arguments for the business benefits of equal opportunities and positive action measures designed to expand the recruitment base did not long survive the onset of the recession of the early 1990s.

5 This argument for a national strategy is not intended to imply the simplistic imposition of a uniform set of 'solutions'. The evidence of our research suggests that different nurse education centres need to experiment in devising local solutions to the challenges posed by local conditions. Even against a general background of

uncertainty and inaction, there were examples of innovative and proactive thinking. We do, however, suggest that a national strategy is required to stimulate and reward action at the local level. Our research indicates that there is a need more effectively to disseminate the arguments for action, to facilitate the sharing of good practice, to promote knowledge about sources of information and, ultimately, to sanction inaction or dereliction.

# Bibliography


Afshar, H. and Maynard, M. (eds) (1994), *The Dynamics of 'Race' and Gender*, Taylor and Francis, London.

Agbolegbe, G. (1984), 'Fighting the Racist Disease', *Nursing Times*, vol. 80, no.16, pp. 18-20.

Ahmad, W. I. U. (1992), 'The Maligned Healer: the "Hakim" and Western Medicine', *New Community*, vol. 18, no. 4, pp. 521-36.

Ahmad, W.I.U. (ed.) (1993), *'Race' and Health in Contemporary Britain*, Open University Press, Buckingham.

Akinsanya, J. (1988), 'Ethnic Minority Nurses, Midwives and Health Visitors: What Role for Them in the National Health Service?', *New Community*, vol. 14, pp. 444-50.

Alibhai, Y. (1988), 'Black Nightingales', *New Statesman/New Society*, 7. October, pp. 26-27.

Allsop, J. (1984), *Health Policy and the NHS*, Longman, London.

Amos, V. and Parmar, P. (1984), 'Challenging Imperial Feminism', *Feminist Review*, 17, pp. 3-19.

Anthias, F. and Yuval-Davis, N. (1992), *Racialized Boundaries: Race, Nation, Gender, Colour and Class and the Anti-Racist Struggle*, Routledge, London.

Anwar, M. and Ali, A. (1987), *Overseas Doctors: Experience and Expectations*, Commission for Racial Equality, London.

Au, S. (1990), 'Bridging the Cultural Gap', *Open Mind*, no. 46.

Bagilhole, B. (1997), *Equal Opportunities and Social Policy*, Longman, London.

Ballard, R. (1992), 'New Clothes for the Emperor? The Conceptual Nakedness of the Race Relations Industry in Britain', *New Community*, vol. 18, no. 3, pp. 481-92.

Baxter, C. (1988), *The Black Nurse: An Endangered Species*, National Extension College for Training in Health and Race, Cambridge.

Beishon, S., Virdee, S. and Hagell, A. (1995), *Nursing in a Multi-Ethnic NHS,* Policy Studies Institute, London.

Berthoud, R. (1997), 'Income and Standards of Living', in T. Modood, R. Berthoud, J. Lakey, J. Nazroo, P. Smith, S. Virdee, and S. Beishon, *Ethnic Minorities in Britain*, Policy Studies Institute, London, pp. 150-83.

Bhopal, R. and White, M. (1993), 'Health Promotion for Ethnic Minorities: Past, Present and Future, in W.I.U. Ahmad, (ed.) *'Race' and Health in Contemporary Britain*, Open University Press, Buckingham, pp. 137-66.

Black Health Workers and Patients Group (1983), 'Psychiatry and the Corporate State', *Race and Class*, vol. 25, no. 2, pp. 49-64.

Black Women's Group. (1974), 'Black Women and Nursing: A Job Like Any Other', *Race Today,* August, pp. 226-230.

Bothamley, R. (1996), 'Issues of Race', *Journal of Community Nursing*, no. 10, p. 10.

Bourne, C. and Whitmore, J. (1996), *Anti-Discrimination Law in Britain*, 3rd. edn., Sweet and Maxwell, London.

Bowen, W. and Bok, D. (1998), *The Shape of the River: Long-Term Consequences of Considering Race in College and University Admissions*, Princeton University Press, Princeton.

Bowler, I. (1993), '"They're Not the Same as us": Midwives' Stereotypes of South Asian Descent Maternity Patients', *Sociology of Health and Illness*, vol.15, no. 2, pp. 157-78.

Bradley, H. (1996), *Fractured Identities: Changing Patterns of Inequality*, Polity Press, Cambridge.

Brah, A. (1996), *Cartographies of Diaspora*, Routledge, London.

Brent CHC (1981), *Black People and the Health Service,* Brent Community Health Council, London.

Brown, C. (1984), *Black and White Britain: The Third PSI Survey*, Gower, Aldershot.

Brown, C. and Gay, P. (1985), *Racial Discrimination: 17 Years After the Act*, Policy Studies Institute, London.

Brown, R.G.S. (1962), 'The Course of Circular - a Study of Reactions to HM(62) 1', *The Hospital*, June, pp. 371-74.

Bulmer, M. (1984) 'Concepts in the Analysis of Qualitative Data', in M. Bulmer (ed.) *Sociological Research Methods*, 2nd Edition, Macmillan, Basingstoke, pp. 241-62.

Bulmer, M. (1996), 'The Ethnic Group Question in the 1991 Census of Population', in D. Coleman and J. Salt (eds), *Ethnicity in the 1991 Census, Volume One: Demographic Characteristics of the Ethnic Minority Populations*, HMSO, London, pp. 33-62.

Burke, A. (1984), 'Is Racism a Causatory Factor in Mental Illness?', *International Journal of Social Psychiatry*, vol. 30, nos. 1 and 2.

Carvel, J. (2001), 'Racism is Rife in NHS Says Study', *The Guardian*, June 19.

Cassidy, J. (1995), 'Ethnic Dilemma', *Nursing Times,* vol. 91, p. 18.

Charmaz, C. (1990), 'Discovering Chronic Illness: Using Grounded Theory', *Social Science and Medicine*, no. 30, pp. 1161-72.

Cockburn, C. (1989), *In the Way of Women: Men's Resistance to Sex Equality Within Organisations*, Macmillan, Basingstoke.

Coker, N. (ed.) (2001), *Racism in Medicine*, King's Fund, London.

Cole, A. (1987), 'Limited Access', *Nursing Times*, vol. 83, no. 24, p. 30.

Coleman, D. and Salt, J. (eds) (1996), *Ethnicity in the 1991 Census, Volume One: Demographic Characteristics of the Ethnic Minority Populations*, HMSO, London.

Colley, L. (1992), *Britons: Forging the Nation 1701-1837,* Yale University Press, New Haven, Conn.

Collier, J. and Burke, A. (1986), 'Racial and Sexual Discrimination in the Selection of Students for London Medical Schools', *Medical Education*, vol. 20, pp. 86-90.

Commission for Racial Equality (CRE) (1982), *Massey Fergusson Perkins Ltd.: Report of a Formal Investigation*, Commission for Racial Equality, London.

Commission for Racial Equality (CRE) (1984a), *Code of Practice for the Elimination of Racial Discrimination and the Promotion of Equality of Opportunity in Employment*, Commission for Racial Equality, London.

Commission for Racial Equality (CRE) (1984b), *St. Chad's Hospital: Report of a Formal Investigation,* Commission for Racial Equality, London.

Commission for Racial Equality (CRE) (1985), *Positive Action and Equal Opportunity in Employment,* Commission for Racial Equality, London.

Commission for Racial Equality (CRE) (1987), *Ethnic Origins of Nurses Applying for and in Training*, London, Commission for Racial Equality.

Commission for Racial Equality (CRE) (1988a), *Medical School Admissions: Report of a Formal Investigation into St.George's Hospital Medical School*, Commission for Racial Equality, London.

Commission for Racial Equality (CRE) (1988b), *South Manchester District Health Authority. Report of a Formal Investigation*, Commission for Racial Equality, London.

Commission for Racial Equality (CRE) (1989), *The Race Relations Code of Practice in Employment: Are Employers Complying?* Commission for Racial Equality, London.

Commission for Racial Equality (CRE) (1991), *NHS Contracts and Racial Equality: a Guide*, Commission for Racial Equality, London.

Conroy, M. and Stidston, M. (1988), *2001 - The Black Hole: An Examination of Labour Market Trends in Relation to the National Health Service*, South West Thames Regional Health Authority, London.

Council of Heads of Medical Schools (CHMS) (1998), 'Action Plan Launched on Equal Opportunities for Medical Students', Press Release, 15 October, Council of Heads of Medical Schools, London.

Dandeker, C. and Mason (2001), 'The British Armed Services and the Participation of Minority Ethnic Communities: From Equal Opportunities to Diversity?', *Sociological Review*, vol. 49, no. 2, pp. 219-33.

Daniel, W.W. (1968), *Racial Discrimination in England*, Penguin, Harmondsworth.

Dhooge, Y. (1981), *Ethnic Difference and Industrial Conflicts*, Working Papers on Ethnic Relations, no. 13, SSRC Research Unit on Ethnic Relations, Birmingham.

Donovan, J. (1986), *We Don't Buy Sickness, It Just Comes*, Gower, Aldershot.

Doyal, L., Hunt, G. and Mellor, J. (1980), *Migrant Workers in the National Health Service: Report of a Preliminary Survey*, Polytechnic of North London, Department of Sociology, London.

Drew, D. (1995), *'Race', Education and Work: The Statistics of Inequality*, Avebury, Aldershot.

Drew, D., Gray, J., and Sime, N. (1992), *Against the Odds: The Education and Labour Market Experiences of Black Young People*, Youth Cohort Study, Department of Employment, London.

Eaton, L. (1997), 'Race Against Time', *Health Service Journal*, vol. 107, no. 5544, p. 18.

Edwards, J. (1995), *When Race Counts: The Morality of Racial Preference in Britain and the United States*, Routledge, London.

English National Board for Nursing, Midwifery and Health Visiting (ENB) (2000), *Targeted Monitoring of Recruitment From Ethnic Minority Groups into Programmes of Education Leading to Registration in Nursing and Midwifery 1998/99*, English National Board for Nursing Midwifery and Health Visiting, London.

Equal Opportunities Commission (EOC) (1985), *Code of Practice for the Elimination of Discrimination on the Grounds of Sex and Marriage and the Promotion of Equality of Opportunity in Employment*, HMSO, London.

Equal Opportunities Commission (EOC) (1988), *From Policy To Practice: An Equal Opportunities Strategy for the 1990s*, Equal Opportunities Commission, Manchester.

Equal Opportunities Commission (EOC) (1991), *Equality Management: Women's Employment in the NHS*, Equal Opportunities Commission, Manchester.

Equal Opportunities Review (EOR) (1994), 'Equal Opportunities in the Health Service: a Survey of NHS Trusts', *Equal Opportunities Review,* no. 53, pp. 24-31.

Esmail, A. (2001), 'Racial Discrimination in Medical Schools', in N. Coker (ed.) *Racism in Medicine*, King's Fund, London, pp. 81-97.

Esmail, A. and Everington, S. (1993), 'Racial Discrimination Against Doctors from Ethnic Minorities', *British Medical Journal*, vol. 306, pp. 501-02.

Esmail, A., Nelson, P., Primarolo, D. and Toma, T. (1995), 'Acceptance into Medical School and Racial Discrimination', *British Medical Journal*, vol. 310, p. 502.

Etzioni, A. (1997), 'Community Watch', *The Guardian,* 28 June.

Field, S. (1987), 'The Changing Nature of Racial Discrimination', *New Community*, vol. 14, nos.1/2, pp. 118-22.

Firth, M. (1981), 'Racial Discrimination in the British Labour Market', *Industrial and Labour Relations Review*, vol. 34, no. 2, pp. 265-72.

Gergen, K.J. (1968), 'Methodology in the Study of Policy Formulation', in R.A. Bauer, and K.J. Gergen, *The Study of Policy Formulation*, The Free Press, New York.

Gerrish, K., Husband, C. and Mackenzie, J. (1996), *Nursing for a Multi-Ethnic Society,* Open University Press, Buckingham.

Gish, O. (1968), *Newsletter of the Institute of Race Relations*, Institute of Race Relations, London, November-December.

Glaser, B.G. and Strauss, A.L. (1967), *The Discovery of Grounded Theory: Strategies for Qualitative Research*, Aldine, Chicago, IL.

Goss, S. and Brown, H. (1991), *Equal Opportunities for Women in the NHS*, NHS Management Executive, London.

Grainger, K. (1976), *Quarterly Journal of the Employment Section, Community Relations Commission,* Community Relations Commission, London.

Greater London Action for Racial Equality (GLARE) (1987), *No Alibi, No Excuse,* Greater London Action for Racial Equality, London.

Ham, C. (1981), *Policy-Making in the National Health Service*, Macmillan, London.

Health and Race (1986), no.5, Training in Health and Race, Manchester.

Herriot, P. and Pemberton, C. (1995), *Competitive Advantage Through Diversity*, Sage, London.

Hicks, C. (1982), 'Racism in Nursing', *Nursing Times*, vol. 78, no. 19, pp. 789-91.

Holloway, I. and Wheeler, S. (1996), *Qualitative Research For Nurses*, Blackwell, Oxford.

Hubbuck, J. and Carter, S. (1980), *Half a Chance?: A Report on Job Discrimination Against Young Blacks in Nottingham*, Commission for Racial Equality, London.

Iganski, P. (1992), 'Inequality Street', *Health Service Journal,* vol. 102, no. 5290, pp. 26-7.

Iganski, P. (1993a), 'Opportunity 2000 Campaign: Enlightened Self-Interest', *Public Policy Review*, vol. 1, no. 1, pp. 30-31.

Iganski, P. (1993b), *Implementing Equal-Employment Opportunities Policies: Racism and Patriarchy in the NHS,* Unpublished Ph.D Dissertation, London School of Economics and Political Science, London.

Iganski, P., Mason, D., Humphreys, A., and Watkins, M. (1999), 'The "Black Nurse": Ever an Endangered Species?', *NT Research*, vol. 3, no. 5, pp. 325-38.

Iganski, P., Mason, D., Humphreys, A., and Watkins, M. (2001), 'Equal Opportunities and Positive Action in the British National Health Service: Some Lessons From the Recruitment of Minority Ethnic Groups to Nursing and Midwifery', *Ethnic and Racial Studies*, vol. 24, no. 2, pp. 294-317.

Iganski, P. and Payne, G. (1996), 'Declining Racial Disadvantage in the British Labour Market', *Ethnic and Racial Studies,* vol. 19, no. 1, pp. 113-134.

Iganski, P. and Payne, G. (1999), 'Socio-economic Re-structuring and Employment: The Case of Minority Ethnic Groups', *British Journal of Sociology,* vol. 50, no. 2, pp. 195-216.

Iganski, P., Payne, G. and Roberts, J. (2000), 'Social Exclusion and Social Inclusion: Britain's Minority Ethnic Groups', Paper Presented to the Cambridge Stratification Seminar, Claire College, Cambridge, 19-21 September.

Iganski, P., Spong, A., Mason, D., Humphreys, A., and Watkins, M. (1998), *Recruiting Minority Ethnic Groups Into Nursing, Midwifery and Health Visiting,* English National Board for Nursing, Midwifery and Health Visiting, London.

Jackson, S. E. and Associates (eds) (1992), *Diversity in the Workplace: Human Resource Initiatives*, The Guildford Press, New York.

Jenkins, R. (1986), *Racism and Recruitment*, Cambridge University Press, Cambridge.

Jenkins, R. (1997), *Rethinking Ethnicity,* Sage, London.

Jewson. N, and Mason, D. (1986) 'The Theory and Practice of Equal Opportunities Policies: Liberal and Radical Perspectives', *Sociological Review*, vol. 34, no. 2, pp. 307-34.

Jewson, N. and Mason, D. (1991), 'Economic Change and Employment Practice: Consequences for Ethnic Minorities', in M. Cross and G. Payne (eds), *Work and the Enterprise Culture*, Falmer Press, Brighton.

Jewson, N. and Mason, D. (1994), '"Race", Employment and Equal Opportunities: Towards a Political Economy and an Agenda for the 1990s', *Sociological Review*, vol. 42, no. 4, pp. 591-617.

Jewson, N., Mason, D., Drewett, A. and Rossiter, W. (1995), *Formal Equal Opportunities Policies and Employment Best Practice*, Research Series No. 69, Department for Education and Employment, London.

Jewson, N., Mason, D., Lambkin, C. and Taylor, F. (1992), *Ethnic Monitoring Policy and Practice: a Study of Employers' Experiences*, Research Paper No. 89, Employment Department, London.

Jewson, N., Mason, D., Waters, S. and Harvey, J. (1990), *Ethnic Minorities and Employment Practice*, Research Paper No. 76, Employment Department, London.

Johnson, M. R. D. (1987), 'Towards Racial Equality in Health and Welfare: What Progress?', *New Community*, vol. 14, nos. 1/2, pp. 128-35.

Johnson, M. R. D. (1993), 'Equal Opportunities in Service Delivery: Responses to a Changing Population', in W. I. U. Ahmad (ed.), *'Race' and Health in Contemporary Britain*, Open University Press, Buckingham, pp. 183-98.

Jones, T. (1993), *Britain's Ethnic Minorities*, Policy Studies Institute, London.

Jowell, R. and Prescott-Clarke, P. (1970), 'Racial Discrimination and White-Collar Workers in Britain', *Race*, vol. 11, no. 4, pp. 397-417.

Joyce, E. (1997), 'The Crisis Ahead', *The Guardian*, 6 August.

Joyram, P. (1994), 'Bringing About Change for the Asian Community', *Open Mind*, no. 70.

Kandola, R. and Fullerton, J. (1998), *Diversity in Action: Managing the Mosaic*, Institute of Personnel and Development, London.

Kandola, R., Fullerton, J. and Ahmed, Y. (1995), 'Managing Diversity: Succeeding Where Equal Opportunities Have Failed', *Equal Opportunities Review*, no. 59, January/February, pp. 31-6.

Karseras, P. and Hopkins, E. (1987), *British Asians' Health in the Community*, John Wiley, Chichester.

Kidd, C. (1999), *British Identities Before Nationalism: Ethnicity and Nationhood in the Atlantic World, 1600-1800*, Cambridge University Press, Cambridge.

King's Fund Equal Opportunities Task Force (KFEOTF) (1987), *A Model Policy for Equal Opportunities in Employment in the NHS,* Occasional Paper no.1, King Edward's Hospital Fund for London, London.

King's Fund Equal Opportunities Task Force (KFEOTF) (1990), *Racial Equality: the Nursing Profession,* Equal Opportunities Task Force

Occasional Paper no. 6, King Edward's Hospital Fund for London, London.

Klein, R. (1983), *The Politics of the National Health Service*, Longman, London.

Kossek, E. E. and Lobel, S. A. (eds) (1996), *Managing Diversity: Human Resource Strategies for Transforming the Workplace*, Blackwell Business, Oxford.

Kushnick, L. (1988), 'Racism, the National Health Service, and the Health of Black People', *International Journal of Health Services*, vol. 18, no. 3, pp. 457-70.

Lee-Cunin, M. (1989), *Daughters of Seacole. A Study of Black Nurses in West Yorkshire*, West Yorkshire Low Pay Unit, Batley.

Leininger, M. (ed.) (1991), *Culture Care Diversity and Universality: a Theory of Nursing*, National League for Nursing Press, New York.

Leisten, R. and Richardson, J. (1996), 'The Ethnicity Question', *Journal of Community Nursing*, vol. 10, no. 4.

Levitt, R. and Wall, P. (1984), *The Re-organised National Health Service*, Chapman and Hall, London.

Liff, S. (1996), *Managing Diversity: New Opportunities for Women?*, University of Warwick Papers in Industrial Relations, no. 57, University of Warwick Industrial Relations Research Unit, Coventry.

Lloyd, C. (1994), 'Universalism and Difference: The Crisis of Anti-Racism in the U.K. and France', in A. Rattansi and S. Westwood (eds), *Racism, Modernity and Identity: On the Western Front*, Polity Press, Cambridge, pp. 222-44.

London Association of Community Relations Councils (LACRC) (1985), *In a Critical Condition*, London Association of Community Relations Councils, London.

Macpherson, Sir W. (1999), *The Stephen Lawrence Inquiry*, CM 4262-I, HMSO, London.

Macquisten, S. (1986), *All Things Being Equal?* Southern Derbyshire Health Authority, Derby.

Mason, D. (1990a), 'A Rose By Any Other Name…? Categorisation, Identity and Social Science', *New Community*, vol. 17, no. 1, pp. 123–33.

Mason, D. (1990b), 'Competing Conceptions of "Fairness" and the Formulation and Implementation of Equal Opportunities Policies', in

W. Ball and J. Solomos (eds), *Race and Local Politics*, Macmillan, London, pp. 45-61.

Mason, D. (1991), 'The Concept of Ethnic Minority: Conceptual Dilemmas and Policy Implications', *Innovation, Vienna*, vol. 4, no. 2, pp. 191-209.

Mason, D. (1992) 'Categories, Identities and Change: Ethnic Monitoring and the Social Scientist', *European Journal of Intercultural Studies*, Vol. 2, No. 2, pp. 41-52.

Mason, D. (2000), *Race and Ethnicity in Modern Britain*, 2nd Edition, Oxford University Press, Oxford.

Mason, D. and Jewson, D. (1992), 'Race, Equal Opportunities Policies and Employment Practice: Reflections on the 1980s, Prospects for the 1990s', *New Community*, vol. 19, no. 1, pp. 99-112.

McCrone, D. and Kiely, R. (2000), 'Nationalism and Citizenship', *Sociology*, vol. 34, no. 1, 19-34.

McIntosch, N. and Smith, D.J. (1974), *The Extent of Racial Discrimination*, PEP Broadsheet no. 547, Political and Economic Planning, London.

McKenzie, K. (1999), 'Something Borrowed From the Blues', *British Medical Journal*, vol. 318, pp. 616-17.

McManus, I. (1998), 'Factors Affecting Likelihood of Applicants Being Offered a Place in Medical Schools in the United Kingdom', *British Medical Journal*, vol. 317, pp. 1111-16.

McManus, I. and Richards, P. (1985), 'Admissions to Medical School', *British Medical Journal*, Vol. 290, pp. 319-20.

McNaught, A. (1984), *Race and Health Care in the United Kingdom,* Occasional Papers in Health Service Administration, Centre for Health Service Management Studies, Polytechnic of the South Bank, London.

McNaught, A. (1988), *Race and Health Policy*, Croom Helm, London.

Meadows, S., Levenson, R. and Baeza, J. (2000), *The Last Straw. Explaining the Nursing Shortage*, King's Fund, London.

Mehta, G. (1993), 'The Ethnic Elderly', *Journal of Community Nursing*, March.

Mills, I. (1987), 'Regional Realism: Reaping Rewards', *The Health Service Journal*, 23 April.

Mintzberg, H. (1983), 'An Emergent Strategy of "Direct" Research', in J. van Maanen (ed) *Qualitative Methodology*, Sage, London.

Modood, T. (1988), '"Black", Racial Equality and Asian Identity', *New Community*, vol. 14, no. 3, pp. 397-404

Modood, T. (1990), 'Catching Up With Jesse Jackson: On Being Oppressed and On Being Somebody', *New Community*, vol. 17, no. 1, pp. 85-96.

Modood, T. (1992), *Not Easy Being British*, Trentham Books, Stoke-on-Trent:

Modood, T. (1997a), 'Employment', in T. Modood, R. Berthoud, J. Lakey, J. Nazroo, P. Smith, S. Virdee, and S. Beishon, *Ethnic Minorities in Britain*, Policy Studies Institute, London.

Modood, T. (1997b), 'Qualifications and English Language', in T. Modood, R. Berthoud, J. Lakey, J. Nazroo, P. Smith, S. Virdee, and S. Beishon, *Ethnic Minorities in Britain*, Policy Studies Institute, London.

Modood, T. (1997c), 'Culture and Identity' in T. Modood, R. Berthoud, J. Lakey, J. Nazroo, P. Smith, S. Virdee, and S. Beishon, *Ethnic Minorities in Britain*, Policy Studies Institute, London.

Modood, T. (1998), 'Ethnic Minorities' Drive For Qualifications' in T. Modood, and T. Ackland, *Race and Higher Education*, Policy Studies Institute, London.

Modood, T. and Acland, T. (1998), *Race and Higher Education*, Policy Studies Institute, London.

Modood, T., Berthoud, R., Lakey, J., Nazroo, J., Smith, P., Virdee, S. and Beishon, S. (1997), *Ethnic Minorities in Britain*, Policy Studies Institute, London.

Modood, T. and Shiner, M. (1994), *Ethnic Minorities and Higher Education: Why Are There Differential Rates of Admission?*, Policy Studies Institute, London.

Moore, R. (1997), *Positive Action in Action: Equal Opportunities and Declining Opportunities on Merseyside,* Ashgate, Aldershot.

National Association of Health Authorities (NAHA) (1988), *Action Not Words: A Strategy to Improve Health Services for Black Minority Ethnic Groups,* National Association of Health Authorities, Birmingham.

National Steering Group for Women in the NHS (1989), *Handbook on Equal Opportunities in the NHS*, North West Thames Regional Health Authority, Personnel Directorate, London.

National Union of Public Employees (NUPE) (1989), *Childcare and Maternity Provision: Implications for Recruitment and Retention in Nursing*, (NUPE Evidence to the Nursing Staff, Midwives and Health Visitors Pay Review Body - September 1989), National Union of Public Employees, London.

National Union of Public Employees (NUPE) (1990), *Warding Off Wastage: The Case For Equal Opportunities in Nursing*, (NUPE Evidence to the Nursing Staff, Midwives and Health Visitors Pay Review Body - September 1990), National Union of Public Employees, London.

Nazroo, J. (1997), *The Health of Britain's Ethnic Minorities: Findings From a National Survey*, Policy Studies Institute, London.

NHS Training Authority (1989), *Equal Opportunities: A Management Guide to the Implementation of a Strategy*, National Health Service Training Authority, Bristol.

Nursing Standard (1992), 'Ethnic Minority Nurses Leave Because of "Endemic Racism"', *Nursing Standard*, vol. 7, no. 1, p. 8.

Pandaya, N. (1997), 'Why Equal Opportunities Initiatives are a Sideshow to the Main Event', *The Guardian (Jobs),* 23 March.

Parekh, B. (2000), *The future of Multi-Ethnic Britain: Report of the Commission on the Future of Multi-Ethnic Britain*, Profile, London.

Pearson, M. (1987), 'Racism: the Great Divide', *Nursing Times*, vol. 83, no. 24, pp. 25-26.

Pidgeon, N. (1996) 'Grounded Theory: Theoretical Background', in J.T.E. Richardson (ed) *Handbook of Qualitative Research Methods for Psychology and the Social Sciences*, The British Psychological Society, Leicester, pp. 75-85.

Ramdin, R. (1987), *The Making of the Black Working Class in Britain,* Wildwood House, Aldershot.

Rashid, A. (1990), 'Asian Doctors and Nurses in the NHS', in B.R. McVoy and L.J. Donaldson (eds), *Health Care for Asians,* Oxford University Press, Oxford.

Rattansi, A. and Westwood, S. (1994), *Racism, Modernity and Identity on the Western Front,* Polity Press, Cambridge.

Rees, T. (1992), *Women and the Labour Market*, Routledge, London.

Rose, D. (1997), 'A Black Mark For Justice', *The Observer,* 20 April.

Ross, R. and Schneider, R. (1992), *From Equality to Diversity,* Pitman, London.

Rubenstein, M. (1986), 'Positive Action and Positive Discrimination', *Equal Opportunities Review,* no. 10, November/December, p.40.

Rubenstein, M. (1987) 'Modern Myths and Misconceptions: 1 "Equal Opportunities Makes Good Business Sense"', *Equal Opportunities Review,* no. 16, November/December, p. 48.

Save the Children Fund (1983), *Stop Rickets Campaign: Report*, Save the Children Fund, London.

Sheldon, T. and Parker, H. (1992), 'The Use of "Ethnicity" and "Race" in Health Research: a Cautionary Note', in W.I.U. Ahmad (ed.) *The Politics of 'Race' and Health,* Race Relations Research Unit, University of Bradford and Bradford and Ilkley College, Bradford.

Smaje, C. (1995), *Health, 'Race' and Ethnicity*, King's Fund, London.

Smith, D.J. (1980), *Overseas Doctors in the National Health Service*, Policy Studies Institute, London.

Stewart, R. and Sleeman, J. (1967), *Continuously Under Review*, Occasional Papers in Public Administration, no.20, Bell, London.

Thomas, R. Roosevelt, Jr., (1991), *Beyond Race and Gender: Unleashing the Power of Your Total Workforce by Managing Diversity*, AMACOM, American Management Association, AMACOM, New York.

Torkington, P. (1984), 'Discrimination', *Health and Race*, Summer, pp. 4-6.

Torkington, P. (1987), 'Racism in the National Health Service', *Nursing Times*, vol. 83, p. 24.

U.K. (1974), *Equality for Women,* Cmnd 5724, HMSO, London.

U.K. (1975), *Racial Discrimination,* Cmnd 6234. HMSO, London.

U.K. Department of Education and Science (1985), *Education for All: The Report of a Committee of Inquiry into the Education of Children from Ethnic Minority Groups*, Cmnd 9453, HMSO, London.

U.K. Department of Health (1989) 'Provide Equal Opportunities or Face a Staffing Crisis, Health Minister Warns NHS Employers', Press Release 89/190, 3 May, Department of Health, London.

U.K. Department of Health (1991a), *Health and Personal Social Services Statistics for England 1991 Edition*, HMSO, London.

U.K. Department of Health (1991b), 'Women in the NHS: Opening Minds Opening Doors', Press Release H91/278, 20 June, Department of Health, London.

U.K. Department of Health (1991c), 'Women in the NHS - Pacesetters for the 90s', Press Release H91/285, 25 June, Department of Health, London.

U.K. Department of Health (1991d), 'Virginia Bottomley Sets Up New Unit for Women in the NHS', Press Release H91/520, 4 November, Department of Health, London.

U.K. Department of Health (1991e), 'Ten Action Points Demonstrate Commitment to Improving Opportunities for Women in the NHS Says Virginia Bottomley', Press Release H91/495, 22 October, Department of Health, London.

U.K. Department of Health (1993), *Ethnic Minority Staff in the NHS: A Programme of Action,* NHS Management Executive, Department of Health, Leeds.

U.K. Department of Health and Social Security (1978), 'Personnel: The Race Relations Act', HC(78)36, Department of Health and Social Security, London.

U.K. Department of Health and Social Security (1987a), *Health and Personal Social Services Statistics for England 1987 Edition*, HMSO, London.

U.K. Department of Health and Social Security (1987b), *Asian Mother and Baby Campaign: A Report by the Director Miss Veena Bahl,* Department of Health and Social Security, London.

U.K. Department of Health and Social Security (1988), *Ethnic Minority Health: A Report of a Management Seminar,* Department of Health and Social Security, London.

U.K. Employment Department (1988), *Employment for the 1990s,* Cmnd 540, HMSO, London.

U.K. Employment Department (1991), *Equal Opportunities Ten Point Plan for Employers*, Employment Department, London.

U.K. Employment Department (1992), 'Projected Trends in the Labour Force 1992-2001', *Employment Gazette*, vol. 100, no. 4, HMSO, London, pp. 176-177.

U.K. Home Office (1981), *The Brixton Disorders 10-12 April 1981. Report of an Inquiry by the Rt. Hon The Lord Scarman, OBE*, Cmnd. 8427, HMSO, London.

U.K. House of Commons (1975a), *Select Committee on Race Relations and Immigration, Session 1974-75, The Organisation of Race Relations Administration, Vol III.* H.C. 33, 448-III, 1st July, HMSO, London.

U.K. House of Commons (1981), *Fifth Report from the Home Affairs Committee Session 1980-81, Racial Disadvantage, Vol II. Evidence,* HC 424-II. 20th July, HMSO, London.

U.K. House of Commons (2000), Select Committee on Health, Appendices to the Minutes of Evidence, Appendix 36, *Joint Memorandum by Dr P. Moodley and Professor Ray Rowden* (MH85), The Stationery Office, London.

U.K. NHS Management Executive (1991), *Women in the NHS: Good Practice Handbook*, Department of Health, London.

U.K. Office of Population Censuses and Surveys (OPCS) (1993), *1991 Census. Ethnic Group and Country of Birth. Great Britain,* vol. 2, HMSO, London.

U.S. Department of Labor (1987), *Workforce 2000,* U.S. Government Printing Office, Washington, DC.

Walvin, J. (1984), *Passage to Britain: Immigration in British History and Politics*, Penguin in association with Belitha Press, Harmondsworth.

Ward, L. (1993), 'Race Equality and Employment in the National Health Service' in W.I.U. Ahmad, (ed.) *'Race' and Health in Contemporary Britain*, Open University Press, Buckingham.

Ware, V. (1991), *Beyond the Pale: White Women, Racism and History*, Verso, London.

Webb, J. and Liff, S. (1988), 'Play the White Man: The Social Construction of Fairness and Competition in Equal Opportunities Policies', *Sociological Review*, vol. 36, no. 3, pp. 532-51.

Wheatley, R. and Griffiths, A. (1997), *The Management of Diversity*, The Institute of Management Foundation, Corby.

Young, K. (1983), 'Ethnic Pluralism and the Policy Agenda in Britain', in N.Glazer and K.Young (eds) *Ethnic Pluralism and Public Policy*, Gower, Aldershot.

# Index

Page numbers in *italic* denote figures and tables
References from Notes indicated by 'n' after page reference